2399

TESTIMONIES FOR DR. BRADY'S
PAIN-FREE FOR LIFE PROGRAM

"Pain affects everything. It affects your job, it affects your relationships, it affects everything you do because when you are in constant pain, everything else is put on hold. I got to the point where I just couldn't move. When I'd get out of bed in the morning and put my feet on the ground, pain would shoot up from the ankles all the way to the back of my head. I went to three different doctors; they ran MRIs on me and all said, 'You have herniated disks in

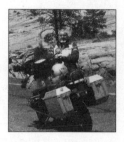

your back. You have to watch what you do. Don't pick up anything heavy. Learn how to squat down to pick up a box.'

"Now, I feel great. People that I talk to about Dr. Brady's program have a hard time believing it. I tell them, 'I'm living proof—you're looking right at it.' I chop wood, cut down trees, ride my motorcycle—I do anything that I want to do."

    —BILL, president and CEO of an industrial supply company
      Suffered from chronic back, neck, and shoulder pain

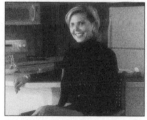

"I was in a car accident six years ago. The pain in my lower back and sciatic area lasted for about five years, until I started this program. It was a constant burning, throbbing pain. I couldn't sit for more than fifteen minutes at a time, so I had to stand up a lot at work. They even moved my computer station so I could stand while working. I wore bedroom slippers to the office instead of heels. And I ended up working part time instead of full time.

"I tried the Mayo Clinic and all sorts of pain specialists. But I was afraid of taking pain pills because I didn't want to get stuck on them. I went to a chiropractor for two years of treatment, saw three different orthopedics, and received a tremendous number of steroid shots.

"Nothing gave me lasting relief until I tried Dr. Brady's program."

    —BRENDA, corporate VP, financial adviser, mother of three
      Suffered from lower back pain, sciatic nerve pain, and
      irritable bowel syndrome

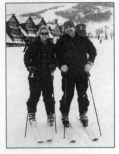

"It started when I was in ninth grade. I came home from school every day with a headache, and the pain got progressively worse throughout high school. By college, I was suffering from full-blown migraines and fibromyalgia pain. I was desperate because I was just unable to function normally. I reached the point where I was open to trying anything. I saw every doctor I can imagine—acupuncturists, neurologists, and chiropractors—and tried every migraine medication on the market. Nothing helped.

"But now, after going through Dr. Brady's program, I live a normal life. I'm not debilitated and I'm not controlled by the pain. For people in pain, like I was, there is hope and there is an answer. It's Dr. Brady's program."

—CHRISSY, college student and nanny
Suffered from fibromyalgia and migraine headaches

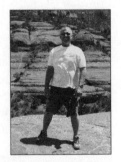

"I suffered from chronic back pain for thirteen years. Some days were intense. There were times I had severe sciatica with the pain running down my back, all the way down to my feet. It was difficult to walk, and I certainly couldn't bend over. Sometimes I had people put my shoes on in the morning because I couldn't do it myself. I'm a contractor with a physical job, and it felt terrible when I realized that I couldn't perform the duties I used to do. I thought about leaving my profession because I couldn't physically endure the pain every day.

"Now, I have a new lease on life. I'm a walking poster child for Dr. Brady's program—I was in severe pain and I am now pain-free. I don't have to hold back, because I know I won't hurt the next day."

—DAN, contractor, builder, and father
Suffered from chronic back pain and sciatic pain for thirteen years

"I had fibromyalgia. I avoided going out and doing much because I had these zinging pains. I became kind of a hermit, even though I'm a very outgoing person. I'm a mom, and I love my kids, so I can't afford to not feel well. I enjoy chasing them around the yard and doing fun things together. I didn't want to feel bad playing with them.

"When I heard about Dr. Brady's program and the success other people had with it, I was a little doubtful. It almost seemed too easy.

"After about a month on Dr. Brady's program I felt great. I wasn't experiencing any more pain. Now, after almost a year, I still have no pain at all! To anyone in my situation: Try Dr. Brady's program."

—CAROL, homemaker and mother of three
Suffered from fibromyalgia

"I've been pain-free for eight years straight. I'm not living my life cautiously anymore, or with the fear of triggering the pain again. I feel like I'm eighteen years old.

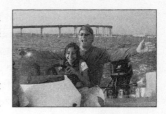

"You start this program and all of a sudden, it changes your whole lifestyle—because you get rid of the pain *permanently*."

—MIKE, salesman and business owner
Suffered from chronic lower back pain

"My pain started when I was fifteen. If I didn't have pain in my lower back, it was in my upper back, shoulders, and head. Sometimes my left hip knotted up, and made it very difficult to sit in a chair for any period of time. Some doctors told me I had curvature of the spine (scoliosis); others told me the muscles around my spine were weak, that they weren't holding the spine in place.

"I love all kinds of sports, and I couldn't play any of them because my back

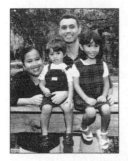

hurt. It was difficult for me to work in the yard for long periods of time. Long rides in the car would cause a lot of back pain. It was stressful for my family when I was irritable and hard to deal with because of the pain.

"At first, I was very skeptical about Dr. Brady's program. I'm thirty-six now and I've had back pain for such a long time it was hard to believe I could make it go away. But now, my life is unbelievably better. I do all the things that I used to dream of doing. Everyone who is struggling with pain needs to know about this program."

—CHRIS, youth director and father of two
Suffered from lower back pain and sciatic nerve pain for fifteen years

"It was hard for me to believe that so much pain could be caused by tension and stress. But after I accepted in my mind that my pain was a result of Autonomic Overload Syndrome, the pain dissolved. Thank God for Dr. Brady's Pain-Free for Life Program! It saved me from having surgery again."

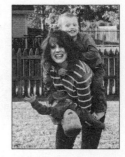

—ANGIE, wife, mother, and computer trainer
Suffered from chronic lower back pain and pelvic pain

"I had problems everywhere—my feet, neck, shoulders, and knees. Everything I needed to do around the house or with the kids required a huge effort. When I was finally diagnosed with fibromyalgia, the doctor told me I would have it for the rest of my life. He gave me muscle relaxants and a mild antidepressant, which made me tired and foggy-headed. Then I was told to adjust my lifestyle and change my diet.

"Nothing worked until I used Dr. Brady's program—it took away the pain completely. Now I know you don't have to be conquered by pain; you can actually conquer it!"

—DEBBIE, family counselor and mother
Suffered from fibromyalgia and irritable bowel syndrome

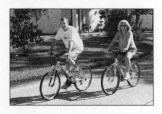

"Each time I went to a doctor for my lower back pain, the treatment would work for a while. But the pain would always come back. Sometimes it would come back to a different part of my body. That really disrupts your life.

"As a pastor, I was intrigued when Dr. Brady explained how closely the mind, body, and spirit are connected, especially when it comes to how the body expresses anger. Part of the problem is that if you see yourself as a good, moral, religious person, you may view anger as an unacceptable emotion. So many of us think that it's not okay to express anger or show it. Instead we keep it inside; we stuff it down. When that happens, the negative emotions get buried and produce physical pain. I'm convinced this was the cause of my pain.

"Now, thanks to Dr. Brady's plan, I'm whole again. It's wonderful. You make plans and count on things that you just weren't able to count on before."

—CHUCK, pastor and father of four
Suffered from chronic lower back pain

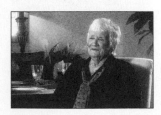

"I had lower back pain. One doctor told me I had stenosis of the back; another one said I had tendonitis; another one said bursitis; another one threw up his hands and said he didn't know. I found doing my housework and walking were excruciating. There were many times I would cry.

"Dr. Brady's program worked in a matter of days. I was practically hysterical, I was so happy."

—ELSIE, active retiree and court volunteer
Suffered from chronic lower back pain

PAIN-FREE FOR LIFE

THE 6-WEEK CURE
FOR CHRONIC PAIN—
WITHOUT SURGERY OR DRUGS

Scott Brady, MD
AND
William Proctor

CENTER STREET.

NEW YORK   BOSTON   NASHVILLE

Credits
General Editor, Florida Hospital: Todd Chobotar
Florida Hospital Review Board: Ted Hamilton, MD, Dick Tibbits, DMin, Richard Duerksen
Illustrations by: Karen Pearson
Photography by: Spencer Freeman

Scripture quotations marked HCSB are taken from the *Holman Christian Standard Bible®*
Copyright © 1999, 2000, 2002 by Holman Bible Publishers. Used by permission. Scripture
quotations marked NIV are taken from the *New International Version®* Copyright © 1973,
1978, 1984 by International Bible Society. Used by permission of Zondervan. All rights reserved.

PUBLISHER'S NOTE: This book is not intended to replace a one-on-one relationship with a
qualified health care professional, but as a sharing of knowledge and information from the
research and experience of the authors. You are advised and encouraged to consult with your
health care professional in all matters relating to your health and the health of your family.

Center Street

Hachette Book Group USA
1271 Avenue of the Americas, New York, NY 10020

Visit our Web site at www.HachetteBookGroupUSA.com

Center Street and the Center Street logo are registered trademarks of Hachette Book Group USA

Printed in the United States of America

First Edition: July 2006
10 9 8 7 6 5 4 3 2 1

Library of Congress Cataloging-in-Publication Data

Brady, Scott, M.D.
    Pain-free for life : the 6-week cure for chronic pain-without surgery or drugs / Scott
Brady and William Proctor.— 1st ed.
        p. cm.
    ISBN-13: 978-0-446-57761-8
    ISBN-10: 0-446-57761-8
    1. Chronic pain—Popular works.   2. Chronic pain—Alternative treatment—Popular works
I. Proctor, William.   II. Title.

    RB127.B697   2006
    616'.0472—dc22

                                                                    2005034003

TO THOSE WHO ARE IN PAIN.
TO THOSE WHO HAVE FOLLOWED ALL THE "RIGHT"
MEDICAL PATHS—
BUT STILL CONTINUE TO SUFFER.
TO THOSE WHO HAVE LOST HOPE
BECAUSE "LIFE" HAS BEEN REPLACED WITH PAIN.
I WAS THERE . . . AND NOW I'M PAIN-FREE.
TAKE COURAGE;
THERE IS HOPE!

ACKNOWLEDGMENTS

I am so thankful and deeply grateful for the confidence and support supplied by my family, colleagues, and friends, from the beginning to the end of this project:

My wife—who has walked alongside (and often carried) me through years of personal pain. Your faith, love, and encouragement inspire and energize me. You are still the most wonderful person I've ever known.

My four daughters—Abigail, Lydia, Sarah, and Hannah: angels, princesses, Daddy's girls. I've missed too many bedtime stories writing this book. Your joy and laughter are medicine to my soul.

My parents—who sacrificed for me, my family, and my education. I am so grateful to you.

Dr. John Sarno—my mind–body medicine mentor. I appreciate you and am always grateful to you for showing me another way in medicine.

Dr. Don Jernigan and Dr. Des Cummings—your strong and godly leadership of Florida Hospital and your vision and dedication to our mission have made this work possible.

Dick Duerksen—your limitless energy and encouragement have jump-started this work many times when the battery was running low!

Chuck Holliday—your message of Grace gave me strength to look at myself deeply—and be healed.

Shannon Sayre and Adeo Media Group—you've been the creative engine behind the Brady Institute from the very beginning. You have God-given genius—thank you!

Many others have contributed to our efforts, and it would be impossible to list everyone. But Bill and I would like to recognize the following individuals for their hard work and support—a reservoir of encouragement that has succeeded in keeping the research and writing of this book virtually "pain-free":

Todd Chobotar—quite simply, without you there is no book. You did so much hard, behind-the-scenes work, but always with a joyful spirit.

The Review Board—Dick Duerksen, Dr. Ted Hamilton, and Dr. Dick Tibbits. Thank you for the tremendous insight, balance, and encouragement you gave on the manuscript.

Sy Saliba and the Florida Hospital Marketing Team—your energy and creativity helped expose this book to many who have suffered; thank you for the great teamwork.

Barbara Smith, Laura Gonzalez, and Lillian Boyd—executive assistants who helped so wonderfully with typing and research, and kept the materials flowing smoothly.

Our agent, Lee Hough of Alive Communications, has exerted his vast expertise in shepherding this project from a raw idea to a publishing reality.

Thanks to the whole team at Time Warner Book Group—including Rolf Zettersten, publisher of Center Street; our senior editor, Chris Park; Lori Quinn, associate publisher, marketing, for Center Street; and Jana Burson, publicity director. You have all demonstrated great faith, enthusiasm, and understanding in paving the way for a book that we trust will free millions from the multiple pains of the Autonomic Overload Syndrome.

Scott Brady, MD
William Proctor

CONTENTS

PREFACE

In creating this manuscript, we have changed the names and identifying characteristics of the patients. But the descriptions of healing methodologies and of physiological, emotional, and spiritual responses of individual patients have been retained as they actually occurred.

First-person pronouns have been employed throughout the text according to these considerations: First-person singular pronouns (*I* and *my*) refer to Dr. Scott Brady and his individual research and experiences. First-person plural pronouns (*we* and *our*) may refer to the two coauthors, Dr. Brady and William Proctor, or to Dr. Brady and his medical and research colleagues, depending on the context.

Finally, while much of this book contains practical, usable programs, *all* readers should employ the techniques, principles, and programs contained herein *only* after first consulting with, and undergoing an examination by, a board-certified physician. Such an exam is absolutely necessary to ensure that you aren't suffering from any life-threatening condition that needs urgent or emergency treatment. The syndrome and treatment plan descriptions in this book are not intended to serve as substitutes for conventional treatments for such conditions as cancer, aneurysms, fractures, vascular malformations, cauda equina syndrome, or other dangerous structural problems or diseases.

Scott C. Brady, MD
William Proctor

PART ONE

UNDERSTANDING
YOUR PAIN

THE HOPE
OF A
PAIN-FREE LIFE

Susan was sitting expectantly in front of me, hoping for a miracle. As her story unfolded during our preliminary interview, I could see why she thought a miracle was the only possible answer to her problem.

Having suffered excruciating back and leg pain for more than seven years, she had reached a stage where she felt hopeless about her prospects for finding relief or resuming a normal pain-free life. Although she was once a vibrant nurse who had literally run about the halls of her hospital tending to patients, her pain had reduced her to a shell of what she had been. Now, thoroughly debilitated by chronic back pain, she couldn't go to work. She was bedridden seven days a week; her husband even had to carry her downstairs when she wanted to get out of bed.

The pain interrupted her rest, to the extent that she hadn't had a good night's sleep for years. All the activities she once enjoyed were now out of her reach: going to the movies, playing golf, taking vacations, driving, or even riding in the car. Her persistent pain had taken her life away.

As you might expect, Susan had run the gamut in her search for medical help. She had seen physical therapists, orthopedic surgeons, acupuncturists, chiropractors, and various pain specialists. Five years earlier, an MRI (magnetic resonance imaging) scan showed herniated disks in her back, and as a result she had undergone back surgery. But the pain soon returned. Another MRI showed more degenerated disks, so she had another back operation. After that, the pain again got better for a few months—only to return worse than ever.

Then came the epidurals (shots into the thick outer covering of the spinal cord) and nerve blocks (injections of anesthetics into nerves to numb sensation). Again, she experienced more temporary relief—but the pain returned.

Seven months earlier, Susan had been evaluated and treated by experts at a leading national health clinic, who had performed another surgery to implant a spinal cord stimulator in her back, a procedure that was supposed to relieve the pain.

"That helped for about one month," she told me. "But then I lifted something, and *bam*, my back has hurt worse ever since."

"How are you feeling today?" I asked. "Describe your pain on a scale of one to ten, with ten being the worst pain you can imagine."

She sighed before beginning her litany of complaints: "My lower back pain is eight out of ten—there's burning, aching, and sometimes cramping pain. And I have sharp pain in my buttocks going down the back of my leg. That's the main problem. On occasion I also get migraine headaches, and awhile back I was diagnosed with irritable bowel syndrome."

As Susan sat on the verge of tears in my office, my mind started racing. Her complaints were obviously chronic, and she was at her wit's end. She had seen so many physicians, but no one had been able to cure her. Of course, she had received several diagnoses—including degenerative disk disease, herniated disks, and sciatic neuralgia. But none of these diagnoses had led to a cure for her pain.

In any case, countless experts had tried to help her but had fallen short. She had submitted to more surgical procedures, injections, X-rays, MRIs, and other diagnostic tests than most people can even imagine. But conventional medicine had failed Susan. Her back was still riddled with pain—pain that had taken all the "life" out of her life.

BEYOND "BODY" MEDICINE

During fifteen years of traditional medical practice—or what I now call "body" medicine practice—I had seen many patients like Susan. Most physicians don't enjoy seeing chronic pain patients like Susan: They're frustrating to us because it's unclear why they continue to suffer, and it's usually impossible to bring them out of pain by conventional treatments.

In my former body-medicine mode, I would have given her the conventional evaluation, diagnosis, and treatment plan. In other words, I would have increased her dosage of pain pills, recommended a fourth round of physical therapy, and talked to her about a newer generation of medications that might help curb her symptoms a bit. Then I would have sent her on her way to yet another specialist—without giving her any real answers or any hope that a cure was possible.

But now I was able to understand Susan's condition differently. Her chronic back pain, headaches, and irritable bowel syndrome finally made sense to me. I myself had once been in almost the exact condition as Susan; I had also listened to the conventional medical wisdom and failed to find relief from the treatment plans given to me by modern body-medicine experts.

My personal path and research had led me out of pain and into a new understanding of the true cause of Susan's problems. Her back pain was not related to her degenerative disks or heavy lifting; the source of her complaints was deeper and broader and involved her mind and body and spirit. Specifically, I determined that Susan was suffering from symptoms related to *Autonomic Overload Syndrome (AOS)*—a term I've formulated to describe the physiological process that results in different types of chronic pain. Furthermore, the great news about AOS is that, in most cases, patients like Susan who suffer from this syndrome *can* become pain-free.

So I spent about forty-five minutes with Susan, probing her physical symptoms, her psychological makeup, her personality traits, and her stresses and pressures in life. We discussed her past medical problems, her family history, and her spiritual history. I asked her about her personal beliefs and spiritual background, because a person's deepest convictions and worldview can become powerful factors in recovery from physical pain.

Early on, I noticed an important feature of her personality that had set her up for chronic pain: her tendency to be a Perfectionist. Susan set extremely high standards for herself and others. Her lists of things to do were never-ending. But even though she put a lot of pressure on herself in her professional and personal life, she usually found that she didn't measure up—and, of course, neither did those around her. Like most Perfectionists, she became irritated and frustrated easily. But you would never have known it, because she had learned quite well how to "stuff," or bury, her dangerous emotions into her subconscious mind.

"I don't consider myself an angry person at all," she said. "Yes, I get frustrated and irritated with people, especially doctors. They think they're always right and they know everything. But of course I don't show it—I'm just a nurse, and you don't tell doctors what you really think!"

Then I gave Susan a physical exam—looking for any dangerous

conditions such as cancer or neurological disorders that might explain her pain. I tested her reflexes and her muscle tone. I pressed on her muscles and joints, looking for areas of increased tenderness. I have found that patients with Autonomic Overload Syndrome often have tenderness in several specific muscles and tendons in the back, neck, elbow, shoulder, and thigh.

During the exam, I reviewed the X-rays of her back. It was true that these X-rays didn't look the same as those of a twenty-year-old female. But then again, Susan was in her fifties. Radiologists had interpreted her X-rays as "herniated disks" and "degenerative disks at multiple levels." In fact, the radiologists were correct in their assessments, but her physicians were incorrect in concluding that these findings were abnormal and the cause of Susan's pain.

I explained to Susan that her X-ray findings would be *normal* in 30 percent of people in their thirties and *still* normal in 70 percent of people as they get older. That is, an increasing number of people have these conditions *without any pain symptoms* as they age. Most elderly folks in nursing homes have herniated and degenerative disks, yet nursing home residents actually have a *lower* incidence of back pain than people in their thirties and forties! In my personal experience with patients, bulging and degenerative disks are normal findings; only rarely are they the cause of chronic back pain. Or as I sometimes tell my patients, "They are common—yes. And normal—almost always."

Finally, we returned to my office to talk.

"Susan, I think I can help you," I said. "I believe that all your symptoms—your chronic back pain, migraine headaches, and irritable bowel syndrome—have a common cause and a common solution. I believe you can become pain-free."

At this reassurance, she began to cry. But these were tears of hope. Her husband, Bill, who had joined us for this final, wrap-up part of the exam, consoled her, but he seemed rather skeptical. I understood his doubts because I had been there myself only a short while before. So I went into a little more detail about the scientific and clinical explanation of the treatment I was recommending.

THE REAL SOURCE OF SUSAN'S PROBLEM

I explained to Susan and her husband that she was suffering from a pain-producing condition that I call Autonomic Overload Syndrome. Here's a simple definition:

> *Autonomic Overload Syndrome (AOS) is a group of chronic pains and other symptoms caused by harmful levels of stress, pressure, and repressed strong negative emotions that have built up in the subconscious mind.*

In AOS, subconscious emotions and stresses build up and overstimulate the autonomic nervous system and related mechanisms— which control many automatic bodily functions, such as muscle tone and hormone production. When these systems are turned to an "on" position for long periods, various physical symptoms emerge—many of which involve pain. These AOS symptoms can involve back pain, headaches, irritable bowel syndrome, insomnia, and other complaints.

Probably the easiest way to understand AOS is to think of your mind, body, and nervous system in terms of an automobile. A car engine is built to travel at moderate speeds most of the time and can generally be expected to last many years without problems. But the car will begin to show a lot of wear and tear if we constantly step on the accelerator and keep the speed at a hundred miles per hour for hours at a time.

Similarly, our minds and bodies usually work well if we keep our autonomic nervous system and fight-or-flight stress hormones at moderate levels of activation for *short* periods of time. Unfortunately, though, the stresses and pressures of modern life activate these stress systems for extended periods. Also, when the pressure builds, strong emotions come into play. Yet these emotions, such as irritation, anger, guilt, fear, and shame, are dangerous and unprofessional to express. So we tend to stuff or repress them to the subconscious recesses of our minds. Unfortunately, though, they are still there inside us, constantly pressing to get out and keeping our stress system turned on.

But I had some good news for Susan and Bill. "I've learned that you can correct these malfunctions of your autonomic nervous system—and eliminate your pain—by pursuing several simple treatment strategies," I said. "These have worked for me, they have worked for others, and they can work for you as well."

SUSAN FINDS A SOLUTION

After I provided her with an individualized version of my 6-week Pain-Free for Life Program (which is described in chapter 8), Susan went home with increased hope and a can-do attitude. During the next few weeks, she diligently applied the strategies that I had taught her—and that you will learn about in this book.

Three weeks later I received a letter from Susan—a message that made my day:

"It is true!" she wrote. "I'm better! I can hardly believe it. I can walk without pain—go down the stairs—and sleep through the night! I even turned off my spinal cord stimulator for the first time since it was implanted."

Then came the best part: *"Hallelujah!* I have so much to be thankful for! I am getting my life back. My husband and I are finally going on a trip—it's the honeymoon we never got to take!"

I don't think that I've ever had a patient who shouted "Hallelujah!" after seeing me. And it didn't matter one bit if that shout was on paper.

After re-reading her letter a couple of times, I sat quietly in my office, awaiting my next appointment and musing over how I had arrived at this remarkable juncture in my life. As a victim myself of seemingly incurable upper and lower back pain, I had found not only a way to overcome my own anguish—but also a methodology to treat patients who were at the end of their rope, feeling hopeless that they could ever escape their pain.

THE ANSWER TO "IMPOSSIBLE" PAIN

The proof of the power of our program in overcoming various symptoms of the Autonomic Overload Syndrome lies in the results of the 6-week Pain-Free for Life Treatment Program. This program has helped hundreds of patients suffering from the chronic, "impossible-to-cure" pains of AOS to achieve significant relief within weeks—without drugs or surgery.

In a recent research project we conducted at the Brady Institute, we studied fifty-five patients who had suffered from debilitating and seemingly incurable chronic pain—all of whom I had examined and diagnosed with Autonomic Overload Syndrome. These patients had experienced chronic pain on average for twelve years. We found that more than 80 percent of these subjects experienced 80 to 100 percent pain recovery within four to six weeks of beginning our treatment plan.

Also, with the passage of time, their pain relief continued to hold firm, according to two-month and six-month follow-up surveys. The various AOS pain complaints that we studied and cured included chronic back pain, fibromyalgia, chronic neck and shoulder pain, sciatic nerve pain, migraine headaches, tension headaches, and the painful spasms of irritable bowel syndrome. Significant AOS-related symptoms, such as insomnia and skin conditions like psoriasis, also frequently disappeared.

Here is a sampling of patient comments that lie behind the numbers:

- An elderly retiree with chronic lower back pain and herniated disks for ten years reported, "Doc, I was cured in three weeks."
- A woman in her early forties, with sciatic pain running down her hip and leg for seven years, wrote: "My sciatic pain is finally gone—I can sit in the movie theater, play tennis, and my husband and I are going to Europe."
- An attorney in his thirties with chronic back pain for three years declared after four weeks: "I'm off my medicines, and I'm 80 percent better. And I'm playing golf again."
- A twenty-five-year-old female with debilitating fibromyalgia for eight years said, "I've finally got my life back. I'm going back to school without pain for the first time in years. Last week I began to have a migraine headache—and I was able to make it go away within minutes!"

Such results in my practice—and also in the work of other physicians who employ mind–body techniques—have convinced me that traditional medicine is too narrowly focused to help cure millions of patients who suffer with seemingly incurable pain. I call today's traditionally practiced medicine "body" medicine because we physicians have been trained to focus almost exclusively on the physical without giving attention to psychological or spiritual factors that influence the body. While I believe that our current medical practice is the best the world has ever seen, our narrow structural focus often precludes us from solving many common conditions. Consider just a few limitations of today's conventional medicine:

- We will soon help the average person to live to be ninety or a hundred . . . but millions suffer from chronic back pain—costing billions of dollars each year in health care costs and lost work productivity.

- Body medicine can replace knees and hips and transplant kidneys . . . but it can't offer lasting relief to millions of people, such as the many patients, the majority of whom are women, who suffer from the debilitating painful muscle condition known as fibromyalgia.
- Traditional medicine can block stomach acid with pills . . . but it can't cure gastritis or irritable bowel syndrome once and for all, so that pills are no longer necessary.
- Conventional medicine can remove brain tumors . . . but it can't permanently cure migraine or tension headaches.

Yet all these limitations often fall away when people in chronic pain are examined and treated with a well-designed mind–body–spirit approach. A new and better medicine will emerge only when patients are treated as a *whole*—with attention paid not just to the body, but to the mind and the spirit as well. Yet it's important to remember that there's really nothing new about this approach. In fact, the seemingly new path I've taken in my practice represents the culmination of landmark pain-related research that has spanned the past century and a half.

A MEDICAL REVOLUTION IN THE MAKING

In the past fifty to seventy-five years, modern medical technology, research, and treatment have focused almost exclusively on the structural or anatomical explanations of pain and disease. Tremendous strides have been made in developing new drugs that have provided a quick fix for many pain symptoms and complaints. But pills that must be taken for indefinite periods are not "cures." Rather, they provide temporary relief of chronic pains that have not been fully corrected or fully understood.

Likewise, once such high-tech tools as the MRI and CT (computerized tomography) scans were invented, physicians fell into another body-medicine error when they concluded, "Anything I can't actually *see* must not be the cause of the pain." Or, even worse, "If I see something that looks a little abnormal, that *must* be the cause of the pain."

But actually, this heavy emphasis by physicians on treating the body—to the virtual exclusion of the mind and spirit—is relatively recent.* Healers among the Greeks, Hebrews, and Chinese have always assumed that the operations of the mind, body, and spirit were inseparable. Also, the ancients often linked negative emotions to physical pain. Consequently, the mind and spirit, both of which possess nonphysical dimensions, were always considered by ancient healers in the diagnosis and treatment of pain.

More recently, we have encountered a resurgence of this ancient mind–body emphasis in the research of Oliver Wendell Holmes, dean of the Harvard Medical School in the mid–nineteenth century. This work continued with a line of other Harvard researchers, including William James, who explored the impact of psychology and religious faith on mental and physical distress; Dr. Walter Cannon, who discovered the stress-producing, pain-intensifying fight-or-flight response; and Dr. Herbert Benson, who identified the relaxation response, which operates as a direct counter to pain and discomfort.

Clinical pain specialists, such as Dr. John E. Sarno, professor emeritus at the Rusk Institute in Manhattan, have developed treatment strategies focusing on neutralizing powerful negative emotions that lie at the root of much chronic pain. At the same time, the scientific underpinnings of mind–body interactions have become clearer with the creative research of Dr. Candace Pert of the Georgetown Medical School, who is a pioneer in the biomolecular foundations of emotions. Finally, scientists such as Professor

---

*For a more detailed treatment of the following summary of the historical background of mind–body–spirit medicine, see chapters 6 and 7.

Harold G. Koenig of the Duke University Medical Center are completing the mind–body–spirit linkage as they examine the relationships among disease, pain, and spiritual health.

My own effort in treating pain at the Brady Institute for Health builds upon the research of these medical pioneers. In my work with patients—as well as in my own personal experience with pain—I have concluded unequivocally that body medicine, though wonderful in many ways, often falls short. As a result, in my practice at the Brady Institute, I've developed a comprehensive mind–body–spirit strategy for evaluating and treating painful conditions associated with the Autonomic Overload Syndrome—the 6-week Pain-Free for Life Program.

YOUR PATH TO FREEDOM FROM PAIN

Your path to a pain-free life involves a process culminating in a 6-week treatment plan that anyone can follow. As you proceed from this chapter to those that follow, you'll most likely find yourself moving through these stages of preparation, understanding, and freedom:

◆ **Evaluate.** All of my patients are first evaluated thoroughly by a board-certified physician like me. That way, they can be confident that their pain has not been caused by infection, cancer, aneurysm, bone fragments, or life-threatening conditions that may be cured by surgery or medication.

◆ **Educate.** Then you'll educate yourself. Patients must understand the true cause of their pain before they can hope for a cure through a mind–body–spirit approach. By reading this book, you'll learn about Autonomic Overload Syndrome—what it is, how it works, and what symptoms it causes. You'll also learn about mind–body–spirit interactions and how they can be employed to cure AOS. The *Pain-Free for Life* material has been designed to promote education along with a detailed description of practical strategies from the Brady Institute's AOS recovery program. In addition to this book, I offer the *Freedom from Pain* video series for the audiovisual learner at www.bradyinstitute.com.

* **Experience.** Next, you'll most likely experience an "aha moment." As you read this book, you'll probably have one of two responses. You'll experience an insight that says: *Aha—that's me—he's describing me.* Or you'll have the opposite reaction: *It doesn't make sense—that's not me at all.* It's my hope that you will in fact find yourself in the patient descriptions in this book. If you do, you'll see more clearly the path you can take to find pain relief. And by the way, when my patients experience that *aha—that's me* moment, a significant percentage of them become pain-free within several weeks.

* **Engage.** Then, you'll engage in the 5-step treatment program. This involves making a firm commitment to embark on our 6-week Pain-Free for Life Program, a series of easy-to-follow, thirty-minute daily applications of the mind–body–spirit strategies discussed in subsequent chapters. As you monitor the steady decrease in your pain—and understand more fully the Autonomic Overload Syndrome behind it—your confidence in achieving a pain-free future will increase each day.

* **Enjoy.** Finally, you'll enjoy your life again as your pain goes away. You'll also enjoy all the insights you've learned about your personality, your emotions, and your spiritual health. After finishing the 6-week program, my patients typically feel that they are starting to get their life back—their pain-free life.

In short, this pain-free paradigm is firmly rooted in the twofold belief that:

* Mind–body–spirit techniques can succeed where narrower, structural diagnoses and conventional treatments have failed.

◆ Mind–body–spirit strategies can help you keep pain-free—
for life.

Now, to get a better idea about how our Pain-Free for Life Program came about—and how it can help you in a variety of practical ways—let me introduce you to the specific ways that it has worked in changing the life of perhaps the most challenging case study that we have encountered so far: Dr. Scott C. Brady.

MY PERSONAL
CHRONICLE OF PAIN

My journey of discovering how to lead patients out of chronic pain didn't start in medical school, during residency, or even after years of medical practice. It started with *pain*—my own pain . . .

. . . Five years of chronic pain in my lower and upper back.

. . . Five years of pain taking over my life—disrupting everything that I loved and enjoyed.

. . . Five years of dealing with expert physician after expert physician—all trying hard to help but not able to offer anything except the standard solutions taught by body-medicine specialists from their own medical training.

. . . Five years that culminated in my midthirties, when the last orthopedic physician I saw said to me: "Scott, you've got the back of an eighty-year-old. You have diffuse degenerative disks, herniated disks, and a dehydrated spine. You'll be in pain the rest of your life—so you'd better get used to it."

At that moment, one path ended, and another began—a new path that not only got me completely out of pain, but also taught me how to help hundreds of fellow sufferers.

IN THE BEGINNING

In retrospect, even though the severe and chronic pain started in my thirties, the seeds were planted when I was a boy. It all started with the personality characteristics I developed as a kid: traits of a Perfectionist and an approval-seeking People-Pleaser (see chapter 5). People with either of these personalities are pain-prone. People with *both* are pain-probable. In other words, it is virtually inevitable that they will experience one or another type of chronic pain in their life.

I have four children—four wonderful girls—and I've observed firsthand how God seems to give every child a special personality predisposition from the womb. I've also seen how the influence of parents, friends, and outside pressures can enhance and magnify these personality predispositions. I've seen it in my own children—and I experienced it myself as a young boy.

As early as elementary school, I remember being extremely concerned with getting things right and doing things right. Although I wasn't outwardly an overemotional kid, I took to heart the innocent ridicule of classmates and friends. My habit was to internalize the hurt—to keep it to myself for fear of looking emotional.

When the pressures of getting things right or being liked by others increased, I often experienced stomach cramps and diarrhea. Sometimes I woke up with stomach cramps that kept me out of school that day. It wasn't that I was consciously avoiding school—but I think something subconscious inside me certainly was!

I think my mom and dad wondered if I was faking Monday-morning stomach cramps, because the pain would usually get better about thirty minutes after my sister had left for school. But I knew the pain was real. In those days, I think the common term for what I was experiencing was *nervous stomach*. And that was just the beginning.

In junior high, I was one of the new kids in school after being sent to a new school district. I didn't know many classmates, and I wasn't part of the popular crowd. To make matters worse, I fell behind in several of my classes. Before long, the stomach cramps worsened—with the symptoms always peaking just after my two most enjoyable classes, gym and shop, and just before my least favorite, English and algebra.

I remember saying to my mom, "I don't know why I get those pains. Maybe it's because I've finished all the fun classes, and I don't have anything to look forward to."

As I would learn much later, that statement was more correct than I realized.

In an effort to find a cure, my parents took me to several doctors, an experience that created more stress for me than anything else. I can still remember drinking a repulsive chalky milk shake for one test. While all the medical tests came back negative, one physician did suggest when I was about twelve years old that I might be developing an ulcer.

From My Bowels to My Back

One day when I was a teenager, my mother, a physical therapist, saw me bending over when I wasn't wearing a shirt. As she looked closer, she noticed that my spine was curved. Deciding that I probably had a mild case of scoliosis, or curvature of the spine, she referred me to one of her physical therapist colleagues, who planted an idea in my mind that would later have a huge impact on my life and my future.

"Your back is abnormal—it's curved," the therapist said, looking at some X-rays. "You don't have pain now, but you probably will. Try these special exercises twice a day. They should help postpone the pain that you'll probably experience later in your life."

Up to that point, I had never experienced one day of back pain. But her interpretation of the X-rays and medical tests, and her unfortunate words, fixed in my mind the notion that my back was abnormal and weak. I actually saw the curvature in one X-ray—there was no missing it. So I assumed that back pain was likely going to be a part of my future. Her prediction of my back pain turned out to be correct, but the cause was not what she thought.

ENTER THE PERFECTIONIST AND PEOPLE-PLEASER

As one who set impossibly high standards for himself—a Perfectionist—I didn't like to do anything unless I could do it exactly right. If I made a mistake, any mistake, I wanted to cover it up or deny that I really couldn't get it right. My mom remembers that I wouldn't even try the hula hoop in public until I had perfected it myself after hours of secret practice in the side yard.

I've often thought that the life slogan for the Perfectionist should be: *You must live with pressure!* Perfectionists always gravitate toward pressure from without, and manufacture even more self-imposed pressure from within.

At the same time, as a People-Pleaser, I was under the constant pressure of needing to be liked and accepted by classmates and friends—and girls. I hated dances and other group events where it might become apparent that, because I couldn't dance, no girls would want to be around me. To the People-Pleaser, rejection isn't just unpleasant—it's *huge*, a situation to be avoided at all costs. When the People-Pleaser feels unliked or rejected by others, the emotional pain is often accompanied by physical symptoms, such as loss of appetite, abdominal pain, and cramping—all pains with which I was intimately familiar.

WHEN COLLEGE REALLY HURTS

These problems intensified when I entered college. My "nervous stomach" had become full-blown irritable bowel syndrome (IBS), according to the physician. I noticed that during the hours before any big test, I'd usually have painful, squeezing stomach cramps and diarrhea that lasted about thirty minutes. Also, I began to experience tension headaches for the first time in my life. The first bout occurred during my freshman midterm week. At first, I thought the headaches had come from straining my eyes when I studied long hours for tests. But an optometrist checked me out and found that my vision was perfect.

"So what could be the problem?" I asked him.

He thought for a moment and replied, "You could try some reading glasses with very mild magnification. That might help."

Of course, it didn't.

My pain story began to accelerate as my college career progressed. In those days, the irritable bowel and headaches were annoying but infrequent, but in my junior year I started to experience the fulfillment of that earlier prediction—*back pain.*

Like most people who experience back pain, the first thing that went through my mind was a full-blown search for the *physical* cause: *How did I hurt it? Where did it happen? What did I do? How did I strain it? I knew I shouldn't have picked up that heavy box! That was stupid to hit the tennis ball that way . . .*

Remembering the scoliosis diagnosis, I thought, *Oh no, it's my curved back! I should have been doing all those stretching exercises— but now it's too late. What that therapist predicted is coming true!*

WHAT I DIDN'T LEARN AT MEDICAL SCHOOL

By the time I reached medical school at Wake Forest University, the symptoms of irritable bowel syndrome and headache had become stronger and more frequent. Also, the back pain intensified to the point that I often had to go to bed with my knees tucked up under me to relieve it. That was the only way I could fall asleep. I concluded that the back pain was from the curvature, the headaches were from all the caffeine I had been drinking, and the irritable bowel was from—I didn't have a clue!

Ironically, even though I was learning about all aspects of modern medicine, I heard little in my classes, clinics, or rounds suggesting that my physical symptoms might somehow be linked to stress, or to academic pressures, or to spiritual health, or to strong negative emotions. After all, modern medicine was *body* medicine. The mind and the emotions were out of bounds.

In one of the first lectures I heard in med school, the physician instructor said, "Two out of every three patients you see in your office will have physical complaints that are actually related to stress."

Wow, that's a lot, I remember thinking. And I also wondered, *How will I know when it's stress . . . and what will I tell my patients to do?*

But I don't remember him telling us *who* these patients would be, or *what* they would complain about, or *how* we might cure them. The professor just left it at that. Unfortunately, no one in the next four years of school ever elaborated on this brief reference to a mind–body interaction. In those days, in the mid-1980s, technology in medicine was booming (with the advent of MRIs, genetics, and countless new prescription drugs). Strict, reductionistic body medicine reigned as the king of medical paradigms.

I realize now that the reason nobody tried to expand upon my instructor's observation was that mind–body medicine was largely uncharted territory. Mind–body medicine was pigeonholed as confusing and irrational by us "real" medical people. The very idea that symptoms could be caused by emotions went against what we considered real science. In this narrow understanding, physical pain could *only* be caused by physical things, such as an infection, heart attack, cancer, aneurysm, or a structural abnormality. If something hurt, we assumed that an anatomical or structural problem must be involved—maybe a broken bone, cancer mass, laceration, or inflammation.

Another intrinsic problem with body medicine was that every physical symptom had to be given a name that had a *physical* cause—especially in the arcane world of insurance forms, which demand a "CPT code and ICD-9 diagnosis." If you couldn't name it, you couldn't be reimbursed!

But here's the problem with that mind-set: Giving pain a name implies that someone knows the *cause* and therefore must know the *cure*. For example, if you've got burning pain in your stomach area, you might have gastritis, or inflammation of the stomach lining. Gastritis is the diagnosis, and acid-blocking pills are the treatment. But the name *gastritis* doesn't explain why your stomach acid is turned up too high. Furthermore, a pill might help temporarily relieve the symptoms, but pills are not the *cure*—they don't turn down the stomach acid permanently to a healthy level.

When I was in medical school, the entire field of mind–body medicine—which today remains in its infancy—was not even on most physicians' radar screens. Mind problems were sent to the psychiatrist. Body problems went to internists and surgeons. Spiritual health wasn't even suspected or considered a part of preventive medicine.

More specifically, nobody in medical school suggested that pain or other physical discomforts might be linked to stress, pressure, or strong repressed emotions such as anger, fear, anxiety, or guilt. Certainly, nobody attempted to link physical pain with personality types like Perfectionists and People-Pleasers. To put this point another way, we lacked a paradigm to understand, analyze, and cure problems that defied normal medical labels, such as:

- ◆ "I've been getting daily migraine headaches for the past two years—and, oh yeah, I'm going through a divorce."

- ◆ Or "I've had a painful back for twenty years though all the tests are normal."
- ◆ Or "Every muscle in my body has ached for the past ten years, like I've always got the flu!"

Complaints about such hard-to-define chronic pain conditions have caused many traditional physicians (myself included for a long time) to conclude that the patients are either pretending to be in pain for some secondary gain (such as seeking narcotics), or blowing the pain way out of proportion. In the end, patients may become resigned to the kind of send-off I received more than once from frustrated physicians:

"Here, try these pills and maybe some sessions in therapy—but you may just have to learn to live with the pain."

Or, worse yet: "Try surgery—nothing else is going to help."

Ironically, patients often contribute to their doctors' frustration in treating chronic, unresolved pains. Patients usually don't want to hear "Your back pain is a result of years of repressed negative emotions like irritation, anger, anxiety, and fear." Or "Your chronic headaches are due to pressure, repressed hostility, and stress."

I learned from personal experience that, like the frustrated physician, the frustrated patient wants a quick fix—preferably a pill that will work fast, and work permanently. Unfortunately, because the large majority of medical problems brought into a doctor's office are stress-related, the attitudes of physicians and patients alike make effective treatment or cure almost impossible. This is why millions continue to suffer from chronic muscle aches, headaches, back pain, neck pain, and irritable bowel syndrome.

And for a long time, that was the case with me.

During my three years of Internal Medicine residency in Orlando, I worked a hundred hours per week for months on end, and at first I managed fairly well. I experienced only occasional bouts of lower back pain, irritable bowel, or headaches. But as the pressures of life mounted—such as studying for Internal Medicine board exams, building a new house, and anticipating our first baby—the back pain and irritable bowel grew worse.

THE FUTILITY OF UNINFORMED SELF-TREATMENT

As the pains and discomforts increased, my intake of prescription and over-the-counter medications increased correspondingly: Zantac for gastritis . . . Bentyl for irritable bowel cramps . . . and Advil, Motrin, and other NSAIDs (nonsteroidal, anti-inflammatory drugs) for my backaches and headaches. Sometimes the pills helped, but they offered no real cure, and the symptoms returned again and again, and stronger and stronger than ever.

So I tried to *exercise* my back to health. I hired a personal trainer . . . lost twenty pounds . . . did exercises to strengthen my stomach and back muscles . . . practiced better posture . . . got orthotics for my left shoe . . . bought an expensive new mattress . . . and slept with a special pillow between my legs.

I expended lots of time and money, but again, I found no long-term relief.

Next, I sent myself to physical therapy. That entailed an entirely new round of stretching and other exercises, along with a special TENS (transcutaneous electrical nerve stimulation) unit that sent electrical impulses to my back muscles. But none of these helped. In fact, the TENS unit actually made me hurt more. (I think I kept it on too long, hoping against hope that it would work.)

Part of the physical therapy involved regular massage. The masseurs identified painful lumps of muscle in my back and neck, which they tried to rub out (or, as they said, "increase the blood flow"). At one point, a 250-pound man, apparently intent on curing my pain once and for all, massaged me by actually walking on my back with his bare feet. Most of the time, the massage felt great, and my wads of tight back muscles would relax a bit. But the pain never went away completely, and the muscles returned to their painful tightness, usually within a few hours.

Discouraged with physical therapy, pills, and exercise, I decided to move beyond the realm of traditional medicine and try using magnets and a magnet belt. The magnet company said that this alternative treatment could help by "bringing greater blood flow to the back through the positive charges of the magnets." I didn't understand the "science" of magnets, and I don't know if any blood flow increased in my back. All I know is that it didn't work for me, and the magnet belt cost *a lot* of money!

Running the Medical Gauntlet

Finally, still seeking relief for my increasingly painful back, I headed back to conventional body medicine by consulting a series of orthopedists and other physician specialists.

Orthopedist Number 1 took some X-rays and diagnosed me with scoliosis. But when I looked at the X-rays, I didn't see any difference from earlier pictures of my back. Orthopedist Number 2, a specialist in scoliosis, agreed that I had scoliosis, but said the pain I was experiencing was too intense to be explained by curvature of the spine alone. He told me that scoliosis usually doesn't cause much pain in adults—and so he referred me to a rheumatologist in case there was "inflammation" of the back.

The rheumatologist felt my back and muscles and concluded, "It's possible you could have early fibromyalgia [generalized muscle tenderness and pain] or ankylosing spondylitis [an inflammatory disorder of the lower back and pelvis]."

She prescribed a strong painkiller, indomethacin, and also ordered a pelvic MRI, a bone scan, and an MRI of my entire back.

The radiologist who looked at the MRIs concluded, inconclusively, that "maybe there is some early sacroiliac fusion [indicating possible ankylosing spondylitis]. But there's nothing definite here."

The bone scan turned up some sort of abnormality in my hip and foot. "Could be cancer," the radiologist speculated.

But other X-rays revealed that, whatever the abnormalities were, they were benign.

As I was running this medical gauntlet, I recalled something I had heard in medical school about the danger of undergoing too many tests. The idea was that if you ordered an excessive number of medical tests, you'd eventually find something abnormal in everyone—but the abnormality might actually be *normal* for that person. In other words, you'd get a false positive result that led nowhere—except to patient fear, more unnecessary tests, and possibly danger from unnecessary medications, invasive procedures, or surgical intervention. For the time being, I was stuck on this body-medicine track, and I knew of no other option.

After the full-back MRI scan—which mainly just hurt my back as I lay motionless in a tube for more than an hour—the radiologist read the result as "diffuse degenerative disk disease." That's one of those diagnoses that sounds official and makes many patients think, *I have a bad back.* But actually, as I've mentioned previously, it's a painless condition that most people over forty have. It's just a normal part of aging.

I then headed back to the rheumatologist, who reported that my blood tests showed an elevated pattern in a couple of areas: "Maybe early fibromyalgia or lupus . . . something will show up in the future, most likely."

To wind up her consultation, she gave me a twenty-minute talk on her holistic thoughts about my pain. She spoke of stress, spiritual health, exercise, sleep, and a wide variety of other fascinating topics. It all sounded intriguing, especially the part about stress affecting the body. But I didn't leave her office with a clear idea about what practical program might help me, or how exactly I was supposed to change my life in order to stop my pain.

After these exams, I embarked on visits to still another round of specialists. Orthopedist Number 3 said, "There's nothing to operate on, so I'll try a steroid shot."

The shot had some numbing medicine in it, and so for a couple of days I felt numbness rather than pain in my back. But when the effects wore off, the pain returned—with no significant improvement.

Orthopedist Number 4 gave me the final bleak news: "Your MRI looks like the back of an eighty-year-old man. Your spine is dry and degenerated, too bad to correct with surgery. You need to just accept that you'll be in pain for the rest of your life!"

"What about a pain clinic?" I asked. "Should I try one of those?"

"I don't like those places because they don't cure anything," he said categorically. "But you can go if you want—I'll write you a prescription for one."

In the meantime, my back pain was getting worse, extending now from my right lower back up through my right upper back and shoulder. Also, it was becoming almost impossible to sleep. On a scale from one to ten, my pain had increased from an occasional five or six before I started seeking medical help to a continuous nine or ten after all the tests and exams.

My back pain even began to affect my family. Although I loved my wife and baby girl deeply, the pain preoccupied me, making it almost impossible to listen well or carry on a conversation. Going out to eat or sitting still for a movie was impossible. I couldn't even toss my two-year-old child up into the air.

The back pain also affected my work, because I couldn't find a comfortable way to sit or stand—and the pain made it difficult to focus on what my patients were saying about their *own* pain. As medical director of the sixteen Florida Hospital Centra Care urgent care centers, I often needed to attend long meetings and listen intently—but fulfilling these duties was becoming more and more difficult.

Even my spiritual life suffered. I remember standing in a hot shower one morning and praying, "God—why have you allowed me to be in this pain? It's taking my life away. Help!"

LOSS OF LIFE'S BASIC PLEASURES

Chronic pain does indeed take away many of the basic pleasures of life—a good night's sleep, spontaneity, and the ability to concentrate, relax, or watch a movie. It makes thinking, working, reading, praying, or meditating almost impossible because, with excruciating regularity, one or another pain impulse takes over your brain. In fact, chronic pain makes it difficult to do anything: physical, mental, or spiritual. I once enjoyed being active with sports, but I became so desperate to relieve the agony that I decided to suspend my entire workout regimen.

This decision to drop exercise, by the way, resulted partly in response to a recommendation by one of the medical specialists I had consulted along the way. He had warned: "The curvature of your spine makes some of your back muscles weak. When you exercise, the other side of your body has to respond abnormally to compensate. That creates more pain and could pull your spine farther out of line."

I also resolved never to play golf again because I had become convinced that the twisting couldn't be very good for a bad back like mine.

Next, I consulted a chiropractor, though this decision was hard for a traditionally trained internist because I didn't know anything about their training. I even questioned if they were "real" doctors. But being desperate, I chose a practitioner recommended by a friend. He took X-rays, examined my back, and discussed my condition in terms that I couldn't understand, using words I had never heard in medical school.

Then he popped my back and hips with some very interesting maneuvers. Actually, I was impressed with the pops. But though the popping didn't seem to hurt anything, it didn't help at all with the pain. I decided that going back to the chiropractor ten or twelve more times wasn't the answer—so I didn't.

Then I shifted to an osteopathic doctor (doctor of osteopathy or DO) who was trained in physiatry—the nonsurgical treatment of muscle pain. He was a very nice guy who was also trained as a chiropractor. His approach was to stretch me out on a table and pop me here and there while he listened to my story. As part of each session, he would also inject a lot of medicine into my back. As I recall, he emptied two sizable, 60cc syringes containing steroids, pain medication, saline, and some other ingredients into ten or twelve places along my back muscles and spine. By the time I left his office, I felt like a pincushion.

Although the shots hurt a lot, by this time I was willing to do anything that might help the pain. I hadn't slept well for months, and I had even more trouble concentrating on my work and enjoying my family. Like many people who suffer such serious discomfort, the pain had become all-consuming.

The latest pain shots made my whole back go numb for about three or four days, but then the pain returned in full force. I continued the physiatrist's program, including shots into my tight and painful muscles, every ten days for four to six months. I also embarked on another round of "manual" physical therapy, which involved regular massage, a new group of exercises, and ultrasound back muscle treatments. But the results were the same as always: some help, no permanent cure, and the return of pain more debilitating than ever.

The DO physiatrist then increased my medications: Ambien for better sleep . . . a new, long-lasting, nondrowsy narcotic for severe pain . . . Vioxx for pain and inflammation . . . Skelaxin to relax the wads of tight muscles . . . and Neurontin, which was supposed to blunt "nerve pain." The only pills that helped me were the pills to help me sleep and the narcotics, which reduced the pain from a ten to a five on my personal pain scale.

I began to wonder: Was this going to be my path in life—increasing amounts of medicine and drug side effects—just to reduce the pain from a ten to a five until the pills wore off? I feared so.

I consulted DO Physiatrist Number 2, who decided that scoliosis definitely wasn't my problem. But he indicated that there was nothing else he could offer in the way of treatment except increasing the levels of medicine in my war chest. He spent about forty-five minutes with me—going through the test results, treatment failures, and future possibilities. I left his office knowing that he, like me, was genuinely perplexed. He treated patients like me day after day, and most of the time he could offer no cure. Only pills and more pills.

Shortly afterward, I made my final visit to Physiatrist Number 1. On this visit, he mixed up something new in the concoction being injected into my back—some type of plant extract, he called it, which was supposed to make the numbing effects last longer. Unfortunately, I had a bad reaction to this stuff, with shaking, nervousness, twitching, insomnia, and generally hyper feelings that lasted a month.

At this time I noticed that my dose of prescribed narcotics wasn't working as it used to—and I definitely didn't want to increase it. This is called tolerance, where your body becomes used to a given amount of pain medicine and then begins to require larger amounts to get the same effect. Although the narcotics were the first thing to bring significant relief of my pain in several years, I knew that the narcotic pain path led to places I didn't want to go: increasing doses to get the same effect . . . doctor visits where the physician concludes that you're a "drug seeker," not someone in real pain . . . and increasing side effects to the medicine.

It was at this point that I finally reached the end of my rope with mainstream body medicine. My own profession had let me down. Not only had nothing helped me, but my pain had actually grown worse. So I canceled all my pending doctors' appointments, stored all my pills in a drawer, and went cold turkey: I just stopped taking all my medicines. Of course, I don't recommend that anyone else should do this. But I figured, what did I have to lose? My physical pain couldn't get any worse, could it? As it happened, I was dead wrong.

FROM BODY MEDICINE TO MIND–BODY MEDICINE

Quitting the pills cold turkey wasn't wise. The side effects of withdrawal are *not* pleasant. In addition, the sharp and burning pains in my back, head, and muscles turned my life into a living hell for the next month. I lay wide awake every single night, my mind racing and my body twitching.

Finally, at the end of about a month, the medication reaction and withdrawal symptoms abated, but the chronic back pain remained. Although I was no longer twitching, I found myself right back at square one. I had begun with nagging back pain that bothered me every night, and now the pain had become worse. It was continuous, intense, and debilitating.

In the midst of my withdrawal experience, my pastor and his wife visited to talk and pray with my wife and me. I was grateful for their concern, and I did believe in prayer. But as a traditionally trained physician, I was still convinced that something structural or inflammatory *must* be causing my back pain—even if God might decide to heal it supernaturally. In other words, I could understand back pain only one way: I gave near-absolute authority to the basic tenets of traditional medicine, based on structural or mechanical pathology—what we have been calling body medicine.

At the same time, my confidence in body-medicine physicians

and prescriptions had been profoundly shaken by my recent treatment failures and conflicting consultations. Thinking of the thousands of patients I had treated over the years for chronic back pain, irritable bowel, or headaches, I recalled with some chagrin my unexpressed skepticism toward their pain:

Come on, I would think, *it can't be so bad! Are you sure you're not faking it?*

Now *I* was the patient—and I knew it *was* that bad and I *wasn't* faking anything. Even worse, no one could figure out the cure for my problems.

A life-changing suggestion came from an unlikely medical source—my mother—who called one night while I was lying on the sofa nursing my bad back.

"Turn on your TV!" she said. "John Stossel is interviewing a Dr. John Sarno, who says he can cure back pain like yours."

I wasn't too optimistic. This fellow Dr. Sarno was claiming that he had completely cured a large percentage of people who came to him suffering from chronic back pain by using a mind–body approach, without drugs or surgery. I suspected he might be a quack, but he got my attention. After all, he *was* an MD—so at worst, it seemed, he'd turn out to be a medically trained quack. But the more he talked, the more I listened—and the more intrigued I became.

Following the show, I remembered that a friend had given me one of Sarno's books, and after a little rummaging around I managed to find it. For the next couple of days, I thought about Sarno's concepts. He believed that physical symptoms might be caused by repressed emotions, including anger. The idea went against all my medical training—but something about it seemed deeply true. His ideas set me on a journey of healing that eventually cured my pain, and led me to where I am today.

PHYSICIAN, HEAL THYSELF!

The idea that my strong, negative, repressed emotions might actually be causing changes in my body and muscles—which in turn resulted in my various pains—presented an exciting new prospect, and a new hope. *If this is true*, I thought, *maybe that explains why no one has cured me thus far. Maybe I can actually become pain-free!*

As I read more about mind–body medicine, I began to explore my own repressed negative emotions. When I did, I could sometimes feel a strange tingling and warm sensation in my back. It was the kind of sensation you get when the blood flows back after your foot has been asleep. Also, my back muscles began to relax for the first time in years. Inexplicably, I seemed to be experiencing the warmth of increased blood flow. These responses caught me off guard. Although I was just reading and thinking, I could actually feel changes occurring in my back! I didn't understand what was happening, but whatever the mechanism, I knew beyond any doubt that something was beginning to reduce my pain.

This experience was so amazing that I thought I must be imagining things. But I continued to assume the role of physician to myself. In the minutes between visits with my patients, I spent time reading and reflecting in greater depth on how my *own* buried emotions might be linked to my pain. The more I dug into my subconscious, the more repressed emotions I uncovered—and the more I noticed an inflow of physical warmth to muscles, relaxation, and pain relief.

Along with Dr. Sarno's materials, I discovered several articles in the *New England Journal of Medicine* and other journals about the link between anger and heart disease, anger and depression, anger and physical pain. But I didn't *feel* angry, and I certainly didn't consider myself an angry person. On the contrary, I considered myself a fairly even-keeled kind of nice guy. The last time I remembered getting really angry was during an encounter with a used-car salesman.

But as I began to explore my subconscious mind not only for anger but also for irritation, frustration, and disappointment, I uncovered lots of unpleasant stuff. Actually, these other feelings were simply less charged forms of anger.

Just reaching down, pulling the emotions out, and contemplating them in depth somehow helped me objectify and neutralize them, turning off a physiological process leading to muscle tightness, muscle spasms, and decreased muscle blood flow. As I "operated" on myself this way, almost as a surgeon cutting out his own cancer, I could feel more and more blood flowing in the muscles throughout my back, reducing the pain. After following this practice for about a week, I noticed that my pain had subsided significantly. If I could put a number on it, I'd say that it was about 50 percent better.

While treating my own pain with this mind–body approach, I began to think about the thousands of patients I had seen in chronic pain. What was I going to tell them now? How would I introduce them to this new path I was taking, a path that was very different from treatments directed by a traditional body doctor?

But before I could hope to help others, I knew that I needed to cure myself. I needed to carry my own self-treatment as far as it would go. In a very real sense, I had become my own best case study. I realized that if I could find a way to resolve my own multiple aches and pains—and if I observed and studied myself closely, recording everything I was doing and feeling—I would be in a strong position to develop categories, techniques, and strategies that could be applied to others in pain.

Although I had a solid foundation of medical knowledge and more than fifteen years of clinical experience, this was all very new and exciting territory for me—territory that extended far beyond traditional medicine. The People-Pleasing voice in my head warned, *Be careful! Your colleagues are going to think you're nuts—they'll think you're not a real doctor. This stuff sounds far out!*

But I knew my colleagues didn't have the answer, and all my training in traditional medicine hadn't provided the answer—yet I was beginning to be pain-free. I wasn't about to turn back now.

My next step to a deeper understanding of mind–body interactions was to take a trip from Florida to Manhattan to visit Dr. John Sarno at the Rusk Institute. So I flew to New York City and arranged to listen to him deliver a number of lectures and observe him as he saw patients for several days.

Over and over, he would ask them questions that I didn't understand: "Why does your subconscious mind need to produce this pain?" Or, "What emotions in your subconscious mind is your pain hiding?"

As he explored possible emotional sources of pain with his patients, my mind began to work overtime. I started asking myself some hard questions:

Why does my *subconscious mind need to produce pain?*
How exactly might my subconscious mind be producing the pain?
What is the physiology involved here? How does it work?
How big is the mountain of repressed negative emotions inside me?
Am I really angry? If so, how *angry? How deep does it go?*
How does all this square with my personal faith?
Does my spiritual health play a role in the linkup between mind and body?

A DAY OF EPIPHANY

Answers to these questions certainly didn't come all at once. I felt like a new medical student—exploring possibilities that I had never considered before. Many of my emerging insights were inspired by conversations with Dr. Sarno and my observations of the patients in

New York who were being cured from chronic back pain, fibromyalgia, or other chronic pain disorders—conditions that were considered incurable!

While most of his patients seemed to get better—more than 80 percent according to one study—there were some who relapsed. It appeared that the patients who got better had two things in common: confidence in their mind–body diagnosis, and a willingness to search hard for strong, hidden, uncomfortable-to-think-about emotions such as anger.

In contrast, the patients who had failed to improve completely seemed locked in a paradigm of body medicine: "My back is weak . . . I just lifted too much . . . this prescription will help . . . the X-ray shows a really old and dry spine . . . surgery is the solution . . . massage therapy will do the job . . . there *must* be something structurally wrong with my back, but no one can find it."

I could hear similar echoes from my own past: "You have a weak back . . . scoliosis . . . the spine of an eighty-year-old."

In addition, most of the patients I observed who had failed with the mind–body treatments could not or would not believe that they might have a mountain of strong negative repressed emotions lying just underneath their calm sweet exterior facades. That was apparently a thought too disturbing for them to handle. They might dabble with the notion that they became irritated every now and then. But a mountain of anger? No way!

My last day in New York turned out to be a day of epiphany. It was time to get out of bed and get ready to observe Dr. Sarno and his patients. I rolled over in bed—relishing a good night's sleep without any medicine—a night free from back pain! But when I started to get up, a sudden, searing pain struck the back of my right ankle, at my Achilles tendon. I tried to stand, but fell to the floor.

A wave of questions overtook me: *What did I do wrong? I must have turned the ankle yesterday without knowing it. How did it happen? Did I do something in bed to twist it?*

In other words, my mind raced to find a physical explanation for this new pain. But then I remembered the new paradigm—*subconscious, repressed negative emotions will cause physiological changes to the body that result in physical symptoms and pain.* These physical symptoms, in turn, can move around in the body: irritable bowel one day . . . back pain the next . . . headache the next. I had seen this phenomenon in a few of the patients I had been observing in New York. Some would quell their headaches with medication, only to find that they developed chronic back pain shortly afterward.

Then I made the connection: *Is it really possible that my brain has somehow managed to move pain from my back to my Achilles tendon?*

Initially, I wasn't quite willing to accept the notion. It seemed almost magical that my subconscious mind would create a new pain to divert attention from my dangerous negative emotions. All my rationally trained faculties rejected such an explanation, which seemed to assume that my buried emotions could take on a life of their own. But I had been exploring uncharted pain territory for weeks, and I was beginning to believe that some of these unorthodox, nontraditional analyses might actually be on to something.

So I decided to test the notion. For about five minutes, I sat on the edge of my bed, closed my eyes, and concentrated on both internal pressures and outside stresses in my life. I also tried to think and jot down notes about any feelings of frustration, irritation, pressure, and anger.

Next, I pictured the physical explanations of my Achilles pain on one side of a mental doorway—and I abruptly shut the door on those explanations. Then I opened another door in my mind leading to psychological explanations of the pain. At the same time, I imagined that the strong link between those emotions and the new pain in my heel tendon was getting weaker and weaker.

I even issued a verbal demand to my subconscious mind: *"Stop the pain!"*

After I sat performing these mental exercises for about five minutes, the heel pain disappeared—completely! In disbelief, I opened my eyes and continued to sit in place for a few seconds. I tapped my foot on the floor; then I stood up and gingerly placed weight on the foot.

Still, no pain.

What was happening here?

I knew from the viewpoint of mechanical, structural body medicine that my "correct" diagnosis should be Achilles tendonitis— painful inflammation of the heel tendon, which typically results from physical trauma or overuse. Also, Achilles tendonitis usually takes weeks of anti-inflammatory medicine, rest, and sometimes physical therapy to produce relief and healing. But I had just experienced an immediate relief from that pain, without any medication!

I was now beginning to suspect that my newly uncovered negative repressed emotions were a window into my soul—a picture of some fundamental things that were unhealthy about my personality and my spiritual life. It seemed that I was being presented with an opportunity to deal with my pain on a much deeper level than I had ever imagined possible.

ENTER THE SPIRIT

Shortly after leaving New York, I flew to Chicago to attend a medical conference. I arrived excited, confused, and amazed by what I had just witnessed and experienced in New York. The heavy anvil of pain that had weighed me down for so long now seemed to be losing its hold, and I felt compelled to continue the great adventure I had begun. As often as I could—for four straight days and nights—

I sat in my hotel room and wrote in a journal, read mind–body medical literature, and thought in more depth about my own stresses, pressures, and repressed emotions. And I prayed.

As I prayed, I explored the Scriptures for possible links that might connect the mind, body, and spirit with my pain. Although the new mind–body paradigm I had been exploring made a lot of sense, I knew implicitly that there was something more at work.

For twenty years or so, I had been a Christian. As with many other people, my spiritual life had seen its highs and lows. During those times that I felt particularly connected to God, I experienced a sense of peace, contentment, lightness, and joy. These spiritual mountaintop experiences seemed related to the absence of any symptoms of irritable bowel syndrome, headaches, and other pains.

But most of my spiritual life hadn't been so high. As evidenced by all the strong negative emotions in my increasingly thick journal, trouble had been brewing beneath the surface. In fact, I began to suspect that my newly uncovered repressed emotions presented a picture that more accurately reflected the health of my mind and spirit than the anatomical condition of my vertebrae. It did indeed seem that I was being given a chance to process my pain on a significantly different level than I would have previously thought.

While scouring the Old and New Testaments, some words in Psalm 38—a psalm by David, a king of ancient Israel—jumped out at me:

> . . . *there is no health in my body . . . my guilt has overwhelmed me like a burden too heavy to bear . . .* my back is filled with searing pain *. . . I groan in anguish of heart . . . and my pain is ever with me. I confess my iniquity; I am troubled by my sin . . . Come quickly to help me, O lord my Savior. (New International Version, emphasis added)*

I did a double take. The passage actually said that *King David experienced searing back pain*! Not only that, but he connected his pain to an overwhelming burden or pressure, and the emotion of guilt. And as he expressed that deep negative emotion openly and turned to God, the inference was that his pain got better!

Here it was—right before my eyes—a connection linking the mind, the body, the spirit, *and back pain*. When Psalm 38 is read with historical accounts of King David elsewhere in the Bible, it becomes evident that he believed that his back pain (as well as other physical ailments mentioned in the psalm) was a direct result of his personal transgressions, including adultery and murder, which caused overwhelming levels of strong negative emotions, such as anger, shame, and guilt. Apparently the problem had been building for some time with the king, causing his health to spiral downward and resulting in vision problems, skin problems, and back pain. But at last, he found the secret: emotional insight, emotional expression, catharsis, and connectedness to God.

I knew I was now venturing into deep territories of my soul—a place I had rarely explored . . . a place uncomfortable to go . . . a place the Scriptures call the heart. *Heart* is the English word used to translate *kardia* in Greek and *nepes* (also, "soul") in Hebrew. The clear message from the biblical context was that the heart (or soul) is the center of our being, the seat of the will and the emotions. It's the essence of our personhood.

A series of new questions related to my pain began to pour out of my mind:

Could my heart also be driving my subconscious mind?

Could everyday stresses and pressures, affected by the condition of my heart, filter through my personality and result in strong, often buried, emotions such as irritation and anger?

If so, might these repressed and buried emotions be causing chronic overstimulation of my autonomic nervous system?

As we saw in the previous chapter, the autonomic nervous system controls important involuntary bodily functions such as breathing, heart rate, blood pressure, muscle tone, and automatic operations of the organs. But if my autonomic nervous system was getting out of whack—as a result, perhaps, of a reservoir of intense negative emotions—that might result in my muscle tightness, bowel spasms, and vascular spasms, all of which cause pain.

So in the end, I asked myself: *Could the spiritual condition of my heart be predisposing me to chronic back pain?*

Resolving to search the landscape of scary and dark regions of my heart that I had never before explored, I wrote the word *anger* at the top of a journal page. I decided to start with my past, which had been very pleasant, at least as far as I could remember. The main memories of my childhood, my mom and dad, and my family were positive. But I wasn't about to settle for these initial, surface recollections. I was determined to get to the bottom of this issue. So for an hour or so—yes, a *full hour*—I dug in and focused just on anger in my past. But when I looked down at my journal at the end of this session, I saw I'd written only a few sentences.

After dinner, I returned to my journal and tried again. I got a full page this time. But for some reason, the word *anger* wasn't opening any inner doors or great revelations. So I switched to thinking about my past in terms of the related emotions *irritation* and *frustration*—which are less threatening versions of anger. Now I quickly came up with four or five pages of thoughts and memories.

Next, I added the words *pressure* and *stress* to *anger* and *frustration* and *irritation*. Although I can excel under pressure, too much bottled-up pressure and stress will cause me to be chronically irritated and angry. Now I had opened up an internal cesspool. Quickly, I was up to ten pages and counting, as I uncovered negative anger-related feelings resulting from pressure and stress (most of which was self-imposed), stemming all the way from my youth.

Then I turned to a consideration of my personality. What was it about just being me that had generated so many negative emotions over the years—emotions that I could clearly see I had repressed or "stuffed" into some hidden space deep inside?

One of the first issues that I began to explore at this stage was my Perfectionist personality. My life had been packed with many shoulds and oughts and rules. My lists for others and myself were too long and usually rather unreasonable. I realized that I constantly put pressure on those around me and got frustrated when they didn't measure up. Life was mostly about getting it right, which resulted in pressure—lots of it.

But I could also see that being such a Perfectionist had created even more pressure on me than on others. I hate criticism; yet I'm my own worst critic. My failure to be the person I expect myself to be creates tons of daily disappointments, frustrations, and irritation—emotions that I usually ignore and repress in order to survive. When I imagined my inner life as being measured on a kind of Perfectionist weighing scale—with the negative emotions on one side and the positive emotions and feelings on the other—I could see that the negatives far outweighed the positives.

This can't possibly be healthy for me—or pleasant for my wife, or my child, or anybody, for that matter, I thought. *How can anyone be physically healthy and pain-free with such an anger-generating, pain-producing personality?*

As I reflected, I also delved into my tendency to be a People-Pleaser. As a Perfectionist, I want to get life right. But as a People-Pleaser, I want to be well liked.

While scribbling in my journal, I began to see how crushed I felt when people were disappointed with me. When my best friend and I had a serious disagreement, I would literally lose my appetite for days. When I felt my wife's disapproval, I would often get a headache or stomach cramps. People-Pleasers don't often say what they think. More than most other people, they have to bury or stuff those strong and negative thoughts—or they won't be seen as nice.

Yet the more they stuff, the more the autonomic nervous system is activated, and they open themselves to physical pain.

As my studying and journaling continued in Chicago, I could already see major changes occurring in my own life—and my body. Dredging those negative emotions out of my subconscious and exposing them to the full light of day was producing an amazing level of healing. My chronic back pain had begun to go away before the trip, and it continued to dissipate while I was in New York. But now, during the intense journaling experience in Chicago—which I have since come to call depth journaling—I could see the possibility of becoming entirely pain-free.

Also, by linking my pain to my spiritual condition, I began to see a deeper force that drives my negative emotions—my spiritual well-being. Although I had always believed it to be true, I now began to really understand how lasting physical health is intimately related to psychological, mental, and spiritual health.

But even as I enjoyed my own progress, I wanted to take the entire process farther—beyond myself to a broader understanding that could be used by my patients, freeing them from the same chronic pain and anguish that had debilitated me for so long.

PRACTICE WHAT YOU PREACH!

During my stay in Chicago, my world had literally turned upside down. I had entered the hotel there with the conviction that I was basically a nice guy, calm and pleasant enough to everyone I encountered. I sometimes got irritated, but I was able to keep it under control. I had left with the new, disturbing insight that I was really, down deep, a very demanding and angry man who was able to maintain a pleasant facade with himself and others only by daily repressing large amounts of strong negative emotions.

As a physician, however, I faced a dilemma. I was ecstatic that my pain was almost completely gone and I was getting my life back.

But in a few days I would be seeing hundreds of patients, some of whom were racked by chronic back problems, fibromyalgia, headaches, and many other types of pain. What was I going to tell them? Typically, I have only a few minutes to see a patient. That hardly seemed enough time to explain some of the insights I was beginning to understand.

Also, there was the question of how to tell my colleagues about an entire array of mind–body–spirit principles and techniques that they no doubt either wouldn't understand or wouldn't be interested in. Being the ultimate People-Pleaser, I found myself wondering how I would handle their ridicule. I had seen this reaction in New York—some of Dr. Sarno's peers looked at him as if he and his theories were from outer space. (Ironically, though, several of those same peers referred their own family members to him for relief of chronic pain.)

Still, I knew I couldn't keep silent about what had happened to me. And when I did discuss my personal experience with my colleagues and patients, I couldn't simply conclude by saying: "This mind–body–spirit approach to healing worked for *me*, but it's too complicated to explain and I don't have a program. So here, take some pills."

The situation came to a head several weeks after I returned from Chicago, when I got a call from several people who were in chronic pain. They had been referred to me by Dr. Sarno because they lived in the Southeast, closer to my practice than to his.

What was I going to say to these people? How could I help them? The only viable answer seemed to be to organize what I was learning, develop a program for others, and then test it on patients with various types of chronic, debilitating pain. So I began to organize my new insights into a practical treatment system.

But before I proceeded very far in this process, there was still one last dragon that I had to slay in my own recovery: the dragon of *fear*. Despite my progress—my pain had gone from a nine or ten to a one to maybe three—I remained afraid that my own pain would come back if I tossed my child in the air . . . if I threw away my medicines, which I had saved just in case the pain came back . . . and especially if I twisted my back while playing golf.

REENTER THE DRAGON

Having resolved to go forward and complete my self-treatment, I put my plans—and my back—to the acid test. First, I went to my drawer in the master bathroom and gathered five or six bottles of various medications I had been saving, just in case the pain returned. Then I tossed them in the trash can, one at a time. The last to go was Ambien—a lifesaver that had helped me sleep when the pain wouldn't allow me to rest for more than a couple of hours.

I'll admit I hesitated, thinking, *Hmm, should I save some of that Ambien just in case the pain shows up again?*

But I knew that if I hoped to be true to my emerging insights, I had no choice, and so the Ambien found the bottom of the trash can along with everything else.

Next, I turned to golf. I've never been a great golfer, but I've always enjoyed playing the game with relatives and friends. With the beautiful courses available in Florida, I hated to give the game up forever. So I had held out hope that someday, I'd be able to return to the links pain-free. This appeared to be the time, but I had my doubts.

Maybe I'm rushing this thing, I thought. *Maybe I should give it another month or two.*

I really was afraid of returning to golf because in the past doctors had told me that the twisting motion helped trigger the pain in my "weak" back. I certainly didn't want to do anything that would cause me another setback.

But again, I really felt I had no choice. So the next day, I headed to a nearby driving range after work. After purchasing a bucket of balls, I selected a pitching wedge, the lightest of all the clubs. With some fear and hesitation, I swung the club and *bam!*—my back tightened up like a three-cord rope.

I've ruined everything! I thought. *I was so much better, and now I've really done it. I've blown weeks of pain-free living. I shouldn't have twisted . . . I should have stretched . . .*

Then I caught myself. Without thinking, I had started to replay those old structural-mechanical pain tapes in my mind, the ones that had been imprinted since my youth and reinforced by practical conditioning, medical school, and the words of countless doctors whom I had consulted.

"No!" I said. "Wait just a minute! My back is *strong,* not weak. I do *not* have the back of an eighty-year-old. I don't have a bad back at all! I've just got bad emotions—a mountain of repressed and buried negative emotions deep in my subconscious. The anger and fear and Perfectionism and People-Pleasing personality are giving me the back pain. I'm *not* going to let my subconscious mind distract me and fool me into thinking that the pain is from golf. I'll do the opposite—I'll focus on the emotions and pressures that my mind is trying to hide."

I turned back to my bucket of golf balls and started swinging, one ball after the other. The pain continued at first, but instead of thinking about it, I centered my thoughts on any anger, irritation, frustration, or pressure that I had buried.

Then I remembered some entries I had just made in my journal a few nights before. I had actually begun to *talk* to my subconscious mind and *demand* on paper that my mind stop my pain. I figured, *What do I have to lose? Let's get dramatic!*

"*Stop!*" I said to the pain. "Stop *now*! My back is normal. I do *not* have a bad back. I have repressed anger and pressures and stresses. I will *not* have back pain. Stop the pain—*now*!"

I was so intent on rebuking the pain, uncovering the repressed emotions, and talking to my subconscious mind that I forgot to pay attention to the other golfers around me. They must have thought I was crazy. But I finished off the bucket of balls, and just before I started to hit the last few, I realized that the pain had stopped. My back was loose, and I could twist and hit the ball without pain. Wow. It worked! My fear of pain from golf swing twisting was gone. So I bought another bucket of balls.

Over the next couple of weeks, my back pain (at that point a zero to three on my personal pain scale) would take one step back for every two steps of progress I made. But the pain was much weaker, and using the mind–body–spirit techniques I was developing, I could make it go away. I'll have to admit that every time I felt any back tightness or muscle spasm, my first thought still tended to reflect the old, inadequate structural-mechanical body paradigm: *I have a weak back . . . I have the deteriorated back of an eighty-year-old . . . what did I do wrong?*

But gradually, I became more skilled at pushing these thoughts aside quickly and going after the real problems. Instead of focusing on the pain and giving in to the fear, I'd turn my focus down, down, down into my subconscious, where I knew those negative emotions were still hiding. And I'd say, *Aha! What's going on down there—what are you hiding?*

Without quite realizing what I was doing, I would exert control over the pain-producing tendencies of my subconscious mind by informing it sternly that it had no control over me. Also, I would demand that my subconscious mind stop the pain production and reverse the symptoms. During this mind–body exercise, I tried to focus exclusively on the emotions and not on the physical symptoms—the old-way body explanations.

THE TRIUMPH OF BELIEF

After only about four weeks using a mind–body–spirit approach, my years of back pain had become a thing of the past. I could now touch my toes, swing a golf club, and throw my child over my head and catch her without even a twinge of pain. I could do practically anything I wanted. And *I understood the true cause of my pain*—the strong, negative, repressed emotions—and that the pain could be cured by releasing and neutralizing those emotions. Also, I understood that my back was indeed normal, and I began to believe firmly that my conscious thoughts and my new mind–body–spirit treatment strategy could triumph over my subconscious mind's pain production.

Essentially the same strategy worked with my other pains and discomforts. The headaches, fibromyalgia, and irritable bowel syndrome all faded and finally left me. I still remember vividly the first time I aborted a migraine headache in minutes with the new technique, and also the first time I stopped an episode of irritable bowel. Now, instead of relying on Advil or some prescription medication for headaches or abdominal cramping, I could stop the pain with a few mind–body–spirit activities.

Finally, I had my life back—without pain or pills. I could hit golf balls without throwing out my back, and I could deal with pressure-filled situations at home or work without getting a headache or a bout of irritable bowel.

I eventually developed a practical, step-by-step program that I felt would succeed for others as well as it has for me. The end result has been my 6-week Pain-Free for Life Program, which has become the cornerstone of the work I've done with hundreds of patients at the Brady Institute for Health at Florida Hospital Celebration Health in Orlando.

Now, to help you embark on this program yourself, let's spend a little time taking your pain apart—that is, identifying and understanding the precise nature of your particular pain.

THE AOS
PAIN CATALOG

At this point, you're probably wondering, *Do I have Autonomic Overload Syndrome—and can I get better with this program?*

You'll recall from chapter 1 that AOS can cause many different pains and symptoms. Yet they all arise from a central problem—an overloaded and overstimulated autonomic nervous system that is responding to dangerous levels of repressed negative emotions.

Now let me introduce you to the various pains and related symptoms that come from AOS. This way, you'll be able to pinpoint your particular kind of AOS pain and begin to understand why conventional medical treatments haven't cured you thus far. In the next chapter, we'll delve even deeper to discuss the physiology of AOS—how the syndrome works inside your brain and body.

THE FIRST THINGS TO KEEP IN MIND

As you embark on the quest to end your pain for good, always keep this in mind: When AOS is responsible for your symptoms, the cure must involve a mind–body–spirit treatment. Pills, shots, surgery, massage, exercise, and pain-relief gadgets may help temporarily, but the pain and related symptoms of AOS will come back until you address the true cause. Then, and only then, can you become pain-free—without dependence on pills, stretching, or anything else.

Also, keep in mind the request I made in the preface: that you use this book in conjunction with your local medical doctor. While most physicians may not understand AOS or the mind–body–spirit link to physical symptoms, you should still consult with your physician before trying this program. The reason is that your physician must make sure that your symptoms are not due to any life-threatening conditions that need urgent or emergency treatment.

Now let's begin to deal directly with your particular kind of pain—by looking at the AOS Pain Catalog.

THE AOS PAIN CATALOG

When the autonomic nervous system is chronically overstimulated, it can produce many different types of symptoms, from muscle pain, to bowel cramping, to skin changes. The main types of Autonomic Overload Syndrome symptoms that we'll be focusing on in this book include:

AOS CHRONIC PAIN CONDITIONS

- Lower back pain
- Upper back pain: neck and shoulder
- Sciatic nerve pain
- Fibromyalgia
- Migraine headaches
- Tension headaches
- Irritable bowel syndrome

- Myofascial pain syndrome
- Plantar fasciitis
- Achilles tendonitis
- Lateral epicondylitis (tennis elbow)

AOS-Related Symptoms

- Psoriasis and other skin conditions
- Insomnia
- Heartburn or reflux

The Name Game

If you have pain or any other physical symptom, you've probably decided *why* you hurt. Whenever I ask a patient, "Why does your back hurt?" the response almost invariably will be: "I must have twisted it," or "I was lifting something heavy a couple of days ago," or "I was sitting in one place for too long."

We almost always figure out a reason for the muscle or tendon pain: "It's pulled," or "It's strained," or "It's inflamed." While these explanations make sense most of the time, I've found that if the acute strain or pull doesn't get better in a couple of weeks, then something else is probably going on. Many times, that something is AOS.

If you've been to see a doctor about your pain, the physician probably suggested some name for it. Don't let that name frighten you! In many cases, the medical symptom name doesn't tell you *anything* except where you hurt; it rarely explains the real process going on.

Your symptom name might be *sciatica, lumbago, neck strain, lumbar-sacral strain, lower back pain, fibromyalgia, myofascial pain,* or something like that. Latin descriptions can sound very authoritative. These names may even sound like a secret medical code, implying that doctors know exactly what's causing your problem and how to cure it. But the names I've listed above simply mean things like, "He has pain in his bottom . . . in the neck . . . in the muscle fibers," and so on.

Although I'm quite sure your particular pain name hasn't been AOS up to this point—since the term is being introduced generally to the public with this book—your medical diagnosis is very likely to be AOS if you suffer from any of the pains or related complaints listed above. What follows is a more detailed look at those AOS pains, with a description of some of the typical symptoms associated with each condition. In some cases, I have also included the number of Americans estimated to be suffering from various problems—so you'll know you're not alone!

BACK PAIN

Back problems are the main reason patients see neurologists and orthopedists, according to studies cited by the *New York Times*.[1] In fact, more than 70 percent of American adults suffer back pain at some time in their lives, according to these studies, and one-third have had back pain in the last thirty days. Furthermore, the costs are staggering: Americans pay an estimated $26 billion total each year for back complaints, according to a study from Duke University.

But back pain is not just one easy-to-describe condition, as my own patients well know. You yourself may be suffering from lower back pain, shoulder pain, or neck-and-shoulder pains—which require a careful medical examination for proper identification.

LOWER BACK PAIN
Many who come through my offices are suffering from long-standing lower back pain—and they are by no means alone: An esti-

mated ten million Americans suffer from chronic lower back pain. In medical terms, lower back pain involves the muscles of the lumbar region, or the five lumbar vertebrae (referred to as L1 through L5), which are in the small of your back.[2]

UPPER BACK PAIN

Upper back pain—which may affect the neck and/or the shoulder (in medical terms, cervical pain and trapezius pain)—is not as common as lower back pain. Nevertheless, it can be just as painful and frustrating as lower back pain, especially when it doesn't go away quickly.

In recent years, upper back pain has become a common complaint from people who work at computers most of the day. The pain commonly occurs on one side of the neck, and affects the upper back and shoulder.

Another common cause of upper back and neck pain is car accidents. Certain types of collisions can result in a "whip" of the neck muscles, causing pain and spasm within twenty-four hours. As is the case with lower back pain, when the neck or upper back pain doesn't go away after a few weeks, the source is probably AOS.

I'm often asked by patients what they can expect when they go in to see a physician with a back complaint. Here is a typical scenario.

THE TYPICAL BACK EXAM

On your initial exam, the physician should ask you questions that indicate "red flags" or potentially dangerous conditions that may produce back pain. Specifically, if you answer yes to any of the following, you'll need an X-ray to make sure you aren't suffering from cancer, bone fracture, infection, or urgent neurological condition of the back:

- Are you over fifty-five years old?
- Have you had a recent fall or direct trauma to your back?

- Do you have a history of back injury?
- Do you have any unexplained weight loss?
- Do you have any unexplained fevers or night sweats?
- Do you have any bowel or bladder problems?
- Do you have any weakness or numbness in your legs?

Once you've been thoroughly checked, and all dangerous possibilities have been ruled out, you'll probably go home with a prescription and instructions to try a heating pad and keep doing normal physical activities. Doctors usually treat your back pain conservatively for a few weeks with anti-inflammatory medicine and sometimes muscle relaxants.

Most of the time, you'll get better in a couple of weeks. (Bed rest was an old solution, but it probably made things worse.) In that case, you can be fairly certain that you have been suffering from acute, rather than chronic pain—an important distinction that doctors must rule out somewhere along the diagnosis and treatment path.

ACUTE VERSUS CHRONIC

Acute pain generally lasts for a few days or at the most up to six weeks or so. Acute pain implies that you're hurting from a specific, definable cause—say, shoulder pain after a four-hundred-pound football player bangs into you with his helmet, or a headache after a brick falls on your head.

Acute pain, assuming it's not the result of some serious trauma, should go away in a reasonable amount of time. In contrast, chronic pain, according to Mayo Clinic definitions, is pain "that persists beyond the time of normal healing and can last for a few months to years." Mayo goes on to say that chronic pain "can occur without a known injury or disease."[3] Chronic pain conditions, including chronic back pain, are particularly frustrating to physicians because they fully expect the pain to disappear after a limited time, but it doesn't. Even more significant, chronic pain is devastating to patients, with more than thirty-five million Americans suffering from it.

IF YOU HAVE CHRONIC BACK PAIN . . .

If you're still having back pain after four to six weeks, you're probably dealing with a chronic condition, and your physician may try to figure out the cause through a number of procedures. These may include conventional X-rays; CT (computerized tomography) scans; MRI (magnetic resonance imaging—you lie still in a tube-like enclosure); bone scans (a nuclear medicine test looking for infection and cancer); discography (injection of a contrast dye into a suspicious spinal disk, followed by an X-ray); and various other diagnostic procedures.[4]

In most cases of ongoing chronic back pain, these radiology tests show nothing unusual, except perhaps some normal aging changes to the disk or spine (herniated disk or degenerative disks). As I've discussed in chapter 2, it's been my experience—and studies have shown—that degenerative disks and almost all herniated disks (except large disk extrusions) are a normal part of aging and are not the true cause of most chronic back pain. If dry and bulging disks were abnormal, almost everyone over the age of sixty (and 100 percent of very senior citizens) would have chronic back pain. But in fact, chronic back pain occurs mostly during the highly stressful years, from ages thirty-five to fifty-five.

THE MRI DILEMMA

When a radiologist "over-reads" an X-ray, that's when the trouble often begins. Radiologists are experts at interpreting X-rays, but they haven't examined you in person to ascertain whether their finding really is the cause of your symptoms. In addition, radiologists rarely call an MRI of the spine normal, because there's almost always something about the X-ray that looks different from the "perfect" spine. Of course, to their credit, since they haven't examined you, they don't want to miss anything. So to overcompensate, they are tempted to name *everything* that might have even the slightest chance of causing your symptoms.

Here's the main problem with this approach: Your body and bones and disks change as you get older. But even if your back MRI has findings that are normal for a person your age, the X-ray interpretation will rarely use the word *normal*. Rather, the report will commonly come back to your physician with a lot of long words and descriptions that may read something like this: "Left paracentral disk bulge at the L4–L5 disk interspace with narrowing but no compression of the L4 nerve root."

In my experience, these words really *should* mean, "This person has older maturing bones and disks—so maybe we should look for a different, nonstructural reason to explain the back pain."

Now, if you're lucky and your physician is accustomed to seeing thousands of these scans and X-rays, he'll look you in the eye and say, "Good news, your back is normal."

Most of the time, though, you'll hear something like this: "Well, it looks like there's a bulge. It doesn't require surgery *yet*, so we'll just treat it conservatively for a while. But don't lift anything heavy or you might make it worse!"

You'll then be sent home with more medicines, a round of physical therapy, or perhaps a prescription for manual manipulation by a DO or chiropractor. You'll also likely go home with fear in your mind that says, *I've got to take it easy*, and a thought that suggests strongly, *My back is abnormal*. Such ideas only serve to perpetuate AOS back pain symptoms.

SOME BAD ADVICE ABOUT YOUR BACK

When it comes to chronic lower back pain, conventional medical wisdom emphasizes such things as poor posture, sleeping on the wrong kind of mattress, lifting heavy objects, lifting things the wrong way, and the "weak back." But none of these things, when changed, seems to keep people out of pain or make back pain patients permanently better.

A July 1997 *New England Journal of Medicine* article reported disappointing results when researchers tried to reduce the incidence of back pain through education programs. The education (a back pain school) targeted four thousand postal workers and emphasized lifting techniques and posture, among other things. The authors reported, "The education program did not reduce the rate of low back injury, the cost per injury, the time off work, the rate of related musculoskeletal injuries, or the rate of repeated injury after return to work." So another back pain myth proved false.

Another article appeared in the August 1999 *New England Journal of Medicine* reviewing the problem of chronic back pain. The conclusion was sobering: an admission that conventional medicine didn't have the answer to the back pain riddle. Or as the researchers put it, "When patients with a simple backache are not recovering as quickly as expected, careful attention must be paid to their social and psychological environment . . . there is not yet proof of a very effective treatment of chronic intractable low back pain and disability." The article was quite correct when it mentioned the psychological environment—and inadvertently pointed to our diagnosis of AOS and the Pain-Free for Life Program.

GOOD BACK ADVICE—OUT OF AFRICA

Another common misconception is that the back is weak and easily prone to structural damage if you're not careful. I haven't found this notion to be true at all. In particular, I'm reminded of a six-month period I spent in Africa (Zaire, Kenya, and Swaziland) a number of years ago, seeing a total of about five thousand patients.

Very few of them suffered any back pain symptoms at all. In fact,

I can't remember treating even one who complained of chronic back pain. Yet as they walked down uneven potholed roads, they were constantly carrying extremely heavy loads on their heads, babies in one arm, and water jugs or gasoline cans in the other. In other words, these Africans weren't following any of the usual Western medical advice about taking care of your back—yet they didn't seem to suffer back problems.

So what was going on there? The short answer may be that they were not overwhelmed with the same emotional stresses in their Third World environment that we deal with in our daily lives. In addition, the African patients I treated were not "professional emotion stuffers" like so many of us who live in "civilized," industrialized, nonstop Western civilization. In their culture, they were generally quite free in outward expression of their emotions.

I remember one day when a patient died during an emergency surgery in Nyankunde, Zaire. The family began to beat the walls of the building and scream so loudly that I thought my life might be next to go. But they were simply being free about expressing their feelings. The mourning that followed was loud, long, and deeply emotional—and lasted for days. There would be no buried or repressed emotions in that group!

AOS: THE MISSING PIECE OF THE PUZZLE

So it's clear that the conventional Western medical paradigm has not worked for understanding or treating back pain. Herniated disks are not the problem. Rotation of the spine is not the problem. Lifting carefully, stretching regularly, and sleeping on a hard mattress are not the answers. All these explanations have one critical error: the assumption that back pain must have a structural cause.

It's been my experience that back pain is indeed a signal that something is wrong—but it's often *not* structural. In most cases, the problem is that overwhelming levels of stress and buried, repressed emotions such as anger, fear, and anxiety have given rise to autonomic hyperactivity. The result is muscle spasms, transient lack of oxygen to the tissues, and chronic pain—Autonomic Overload Syndrome. The great news, for many sufferers of chronic back pain, is that the Pain-Free for Life Program addresses the very roots of AOS so that you can reverse the problem and make the pain disappear once and for all.

SCIATIC NERVE PAIN

Sciatica is a problem that often begins with lower back pain and then radiates downward along the sciatic nerve. Sciatica (sciatic nerve pain) symptoms cause pain anywhere along the sciatic nerve path. Areas affected may include the groin, buttocks, thigh, back of the leg, or even foot. There is frequently tenderness when you touch the sciatic notch—the area in the midbuttocks where the sciatic nerve comes out of the spine and begins its path down the leg.

Sciatic nerve pain is often described as "burning," or "hurting like a toothache." It hurts even more when pressure is put on the sciatic nerve, as would happen if you sat down for a while on a hard surface. Conversely, standing often alleviates the pain temporarily. According to the National Institute of Neurological Disorders and Stroke (National Institutes of Health), the conventional medical explanations for sciatica include exertion, obesity, herniated disk, and poor posture, all of which can place pressure on the sciatic nerve.

It's been my experience, however, that many seemingly normal patients—who are thin, have good posture, and have not lifted extremely heavy objects—*still* suffer from sciatica. In addition, sciatic nerve pain not only can occur in the *absence* of any disk abnormalities, but can also arise when there *is* a disk problem. In other words, conventional body-medicine diagnoses come up short with certain types of sciatica. But the Pain-Free for Life Program can frequently identify and alleviate these "mysterious" sciatic nerve symptoms altogether.

FIBROMYALGIA

Four to six million Americans suffer from fibromyalgia, and the numbers are increasing. More than ten thousand medical articles have addressed fibromyalgia in the past ten years, yet conventional medical treatments still offer no cure. Women in particular suffer from this condition: About 80 percent of those affected are female.[5]

Fibromyalgia patients suffer from a wide array of symptoms: chronic widespread pain for at least three months; fatigue; tender points; and the presence of other medical conditions such as irritable bowel syndrome, headaches, and sleep disturbances. Most of the time, fibromyalgia sufferers have tenderness in about a dozen areas of the body (tender points). One of my AOS patients with fibromyalgia describes her symptoms this way: "It feels like you've got the flu a lot of the time. You're exhausted, and if one thing isn't hurting you, another thing will."

This painful condition often affects muscles of the back, neck, legs, hips, shoulders, and hands; however, there are no boundaries. The muscle pain often migrates all over the body and is commonly described as "deep aching, throbbing, stabbing, or shooting." The pain is often worse in the morning; the symptoms also seem to get worse after having a poor night's sleep, undergoing a stressful situation, or overexerting yourself physically.

The cause of fibromyalgia has remained a mystery to modern medicine. Although there have been some hints of physiological abnormalities and genetic predisposition, no smoking gun of causation has been found. Some have suggested that fibromyalgia may be triggered by a viral or bacterial infection, a traumatic event (such as an auto accident), or a serious illness. Yet in the end, it is amazing how very little medical science actually knows about the cause or the cure for fibromyalgia.

After reflecting on my clinical experience with fibromyalgia patients, I am inclined to agree with those studies that say the most likely cause can be traced to negative and repressed emotions, such as anger and anxiety, which may stimulate or aggravate the pain.[6] In my opinion, then, fibromyalgia is a severe but treatable form of AOS. Fibromyalgia sufferers who have gone through the Pain-Free Program often experience significant and lasting pain relief.

HEADACHES

About forty-five million Americans suffer from headaches, including tension headaches and migraines. Various studies have linked these complaints to poorly managed stress and psychosomatic (mind–body) illness.[7] The most common types of AOS chronic headache are migraines and tension headaches.

MIGRAINES
These severe headaches, which afflict an estimated twenty-eight million Americans,[8] are caused by blood vessel constriction (narrowing) followed by blood vessel dilation (swelling). The pain of a migraine headache is usually intense, and may involve:

- Throbbing ache on one or both sides of the head.
- Nausea or vomiting.
- Photophobia (being bothered by light).
- Feeling tired or confused.
- Vision disturbances.

The classic migraine begins with a warning sign, or aura. Most of the time, the aura is a visual disturbance, including a flash of light or blind spot in the visual field. Not all auras are visual, however: They may involve a tingling or prickly sensation just before the migraine begins or at the same time as the headache.

Another type of migraine, the common migraine, doesn't begin with an aura. Common migraines usually occur only on one side of the head, and they last longer than the classic migraine—to the point that they interfere with daily activities. These headaches may disable a person for hours or days.

In the past ten years, many helpful medications for migraines have hit the market. Still, a nagging question remains in my mind: What causes the blood vessels to constrict and dilate in the first place?

In answer, I believe that repressed emotions in the subconscious mind cause autonomic nervous system activation, which leads to the blood vessel changes in migraine headaches—or AOS.

TENSION HEADACHES

These are the most common type of headaches and can often be linked directly to some outside pressure or stress. Tension headaches are characterized by a constant dull, achy feeling on both sides of the head. Sometimes patients have said that they feel an extremely tight band has been wrapped around their head.[9]

Tension headaches are also called stress headaches. Most of the time, they are treated with over-the-counter medicines, a heating pad on the neck, extra sleep, or taking a break from the stressful events of the day. In my practice at the Brady Institute, patients with chronic recurring tension headaches have had great success with the Pain-Free for Life Program because the real culprit is usually Autonomic Overload Syndrome.

Irritable Bowel Syndrome (IBS)

Approximately 10 to 15 percent of people in North America suffer from irritable bowel syndrome, which may be characterized by bloating, diarrhea or constipation, and painful abdominal cramps that usually go away after a bowel movement. The disease affects three times as many women as men and accounts for 12 percent of all visits to primary care physicians.[10] Also, IBS often accompanies other symptoms of AOS, including fibromyalgia. IBS is also called irritable colon and spastic colon.

IBS was once called functional bowel syndrome—meaning that there was thought to be a psychological or emotional component to symptom development. In a 1998 study published by *Gut*, researchers studied 166 IBS patients over a sixteen-month period. Of those patients who improved, none had a significant stressful event or stressor (such as divorce, relationship issues, lawsuits, or business failure) during the study. On the other hand, researchers said, the presence of at least one significant stressor "highly predicted symptom intensity."

Treatments for IBS usually focus on eating fiber, avoiding foods that make you feel worse, taking pills to help relax the intestines, and finding ways to manage your stress. Still, such treatments don't answer some basic questions: *Why do my bowels squeeze abnormally? What causes it in the first place? Will finding the cause enable me to discover a treatment and stop having IBS altogether?*

In my practice, IBS, which is just another expression of AOS, has responded extremely well to the Pain-Free for Life Program.

Myofascial Pain Syndrome

This condition involves irritation of the muscles and muscle-covering tissue of the back and neck[11]—but it is not linked to any physical abnormality or disease. Rather, the cause typically involves a stressful response to negative emotions.[12] In some classifications, myofascial pain conditions are said to include muscle tension headaches, soft tissue pain in the neck, and regional shoulder pain, all of which may be linked to Autonomic Overload Syndrome.

According to a May 2003 report from NIAMS, the arthritic and muscular pain specialists at the National Institutes of Health, the cause of myofascial pain syndrome is "unknown." What *is* known is that this pain affects sensitive areas in the body's muscles known as trigger points.

Various scientific studies have reported a number of possibly helpful treatments, including biofeedback (a training procedure to increase control over autonomic responses) and certain drugs. But researchers have found that behavioral techniques have been as successful as biofeedback in treating those myofascial pain syndromes that are mediated by the sympathetic nervous system (part of the autonomic nervous system). These behavioral techniques, designed to stimulate the "relaxing" parasympathetic nervous system, include relaxation training (including word-focus techniques to elicit the relaxation response), autogenic training (passive focus on bodily sensations), and progressive muscle relaxation.

The problem with drug-related treatments is that they do not constitute a cure if you have to take a particular pill over and over again. The program you'll read about in part 2 of this book is designed to turn down the overloaded autonomic nervous system and stop AOS symptoms (including myofascial pain) altogether—but without drugs or invasive medical procedures.

PLANTAR FASCIITIS

The plantar fascia is a band of tissue on the bottom of your foot; it starts at your heel and attaches to little bones at the ball of your foot. Plantar fasciitis, a common cause of heel pain, is thought to involve inflammation or irritation of the fascia. Those suffering from this problem typically feel pain when they walk on the affected foot or when certain parts of the heel or bottom of the foot are touched or pressed.

Most patients with plantar fasciitis explain their pain as "feeling like a knife sticking into my heel," or into the bottom of the foot. Standing for extended periods of time or walking on hard surfaces may aggravate the symptoms.

Traditional treatments have focused on stretching exercises, staying off the foot for a while, wearing arch supports, and taking anti-inflammatory pills. But this complaint, like the other pains in the Autonomic Overload Syndrome list, responds well to the Pain-Free for Life Program, which is described in detail beginning in chapter 8.

TENDONITIS CONDITIONS

Various AOS-related tendonitis conditions, which involve pains arising from various tendons in the body, can also be successfully treated with the Pain-Free for Life Program treatments. Two complaints of this type that I have had considerable success treating are tennis elbow and Achilles tendonitis.

TENNIS ELBOW

This condition, technically known as lateral epicondylitis, has been labeled "tennis elbow" because it afflicts many tennis players. It usually involves pains that radiate from the outer elbow (epicondyle) down through the tendons on the upper side of the forearm. The pain becomes especially sharp when the patient tries to grasp or twist something with the hand—opening the tight lid of a jar, for instance, or attempting to swing or rotate an object such as a tennis racket. These pains are frequently treated with rest, ice, a tight band around the muscles of the upper forearm, and anti-inflammatory medications.

ACHILLES TENDONITIS

This problem refers to a severe pain and soreness of the large, ropey tendon at the back of the heel—the Achilles tendon. It's thought to be caused by abnormal physical strain, which results in inflammation. Normal inflammation, however, usually subsides with rest in seven to ten days; Achilles tendonitis can last for months. When the problem persists for long periods of time, I usually treat it as an AOS condition (my pain story in chapter 2 provides an illustration).

AUTONOMIC OVERLOAD SYNDROME–RELATED CONDITIONS

AOS produces pain in most cases. However, autonomic activation can produce other, nonpainful symptoms as well. As I've observed many patients with AOS pain conditions achieving pain relief through the Pain-Free Program, I have also noted that other symptoms, such as the following, may frequently improve.

PSORIASIS AND OTHER SKIN IRRITATIONS

Stress and negative thoughts and emotions are major factors in triggering skin conditions. The most common of these skin problems are adult acne, psoriasis, rosacea, and eczema. Both inception and aggravation of these conditions has been associated with repressed emotions.[13]

The *Archives of Dermatology* published a report in 1998 that said, "stress and negative thoughts are major factors in dermatologic (skin) conditions. . . . Mind–body interventions can improve dermatologic conditions and, in most cases, quality of life."[14]

Dr. Jon Kabat-Zinn from the University of Massachusetts has had wonderful success treating psoriasis with a mind–body intervention called mindfulness meditation. In 1998, he published an article reporting that meditation and relaxation techniques were able to improve psoriasis by 50 percent.[15]

One of the first patients I ever treated with the Pain-Free Program suffered from chronic back pain and plantar fasciitis. When I called him a couple of weeks after his exam to see how he was getting along, to my surprise he said, "I can't believe it, my psoriasis is completely gone, I've had it for twenty years."

I was taken aback because his main problem was chronic back pain, for more than a decade. So I asked again about his back and he replied, "Oh yeah, that's getting better and I've already played golf once. But you wouldn't believe my skin, I look great."

INSOMNIA

A good night's sleep is wonderful—and, too often, rare. An estimated twenty-two million people experience the torment of chronic insomnia. Insomnia can assume different faces, including difficulty falling asleep, waking up frequently during the night with trouble getting back to sleep, waking up too early in the morning, and experiencing generally unrefreshing sleep.

There are many reasons for insomnia, among them the use of stimulants like caffeine, poorly managed stress, smoking, and the side effects of many medications. Also, insomnia can be caused by sleep disrupters, such as snoring, sleep apnea, jet lag, and environmental noise. Insomnia seems to be more common among those who are female, who have a history of depression, and who are older.

Many AOS patients complain of insomnia in addition to their chronic pain. Sometimes the pain itself makes it difficult to sleep. Other times, even though patients don't have any pain at night, they just don't sleep well.

The treatment for chronic insomnia varies depending on the cause. In general, if there are no medical problems (such as sleep apnea), the treatment will include identifying and reducing the things that overstimulate the brain; trying behavioral techniques like relaxation therapy; and, sometimes, embarking on a short course of medication (but this strategy is controversial, even among many physicians who focus on body medicine).

In my practice, I've found that the combination of stopping brain-stimulating caffeine and nicotine, and changing medications that have stimulating side effects—along with starting the stress-busting, repressed-emotion-uncovering Pain-Free for Life Program—often helps AOS patients get a good night's sleep.

HEARTBURN (REFLUX)

Heartburn is a burning sensation in the lower middle chest just below the ribs. Like all medical symptoms, heartburn can be a sign of a serious medical condition, such as a heart attack, abdominal aneurysm, esophageal cancer, or ulcers, to name a few possibilities. So your local doctor should check you thoroughly before you decide to diagnose and treat yourself with antacids.

Once the dangerous options are ruled out, you will probably find that you are dealing with the very common condition of heartburn, otherwise known as GERD (gastroesophageal reflux disease).

Heartburn symptoms occur when excessive stomach acid is produced and enters the opening—which should be closed—between your stomach and esophagus. GERD symptoms can be made worse by such factors as smoking, drinking coffee or alcohol, eating citrus fruits, taking aspirin, being overweight, or consuming lots of caffeine-laden sodas or chocolate. Most of the time, heartburn can be relieved with antacids or over-the-counter H2 blockers like Zantac, Pepcid, and Tagamet, which turn off the acid-making machine. If these treatments don't work, many physicians will prescribe stronger pills and recommend an endoscopy (a procedure employing a little camera that enables a specialist to look down your esophagus into your stomach).

But despite the wonderful medications and scopes used to diagnose and treat GERD, questions often remain in your mind: *Why does my stomach really produce too much acid? Is my diet the only reason the acid is leaking back into the esophagus? Will stronger medications really help—and are they necessary?*

I've found in my practice that the assumptions behind such questions may be off base. In fact, Autonomic Overload Syndrome may contribute significantly to changes in stomach acid production, which leads to heartburn. When this is the case, the Pain-Free for Life Program has proven effective to help this AOS symptom.

HOW THE SCIENCE WORKS IN PRACTICE: AN AOS STUDY

While the above symptom list is not exhaustive, these are the most common problems I've seen in my practice with AOS patients. In addition, these symptoms have all responded well to the Pain-Free for Life Program. In fact, a few years ago I was asked to quantify the benefits of the program for my patients—so in 2000, I conducted an eight-month prospective study on patients I had diagnosed with Autonomic Overload Syndrome at the Brady Institute for Health.* Of fifty-five consecutive patients I examined for this project, fifty were diagnosed with AOS. On average, the patients had experienced chronic pain for a little more than seven years. Their primary pain complaints were:

---

* *Note:* The diagnosis of AOS should be made by a medical doctor with expertise in mind–body medicine and knowledge of either Autonomic Overload Syndrome or Tension Myositis Syndrome.

- Chronic lower back pain (25 patients).
- Chronic neck and shoulder pain (10 patients).
- Fibromyalgia (10 patients).
- Sciatic neuralgia (3 patients).
- Myofascial pain syndrome (2 patients).

In addition to these primary pain symptoms, 80 percent of the group had at least one of the following AOS-related symptoms— and some had multiple symptoms:

- Headaches (tension and migraine) (23 patients).
- Gastritis or reflux (19 patients).
- Irritable bowel syndrome (13 patients).
- Insomnia (13 patients).
- Eczema or psoriasis (5 patients).

All fifty patients met the following criteria for the diagnosis of AOS:

- AOS-type pain and pain-related symptoms (described above).
- An AOS pain-prone personality.
- Absence of cancer, infection, fracture, aneurysm, emergent neurological disorder, or obvious structural abnormality.
- Tenderness in at least one of the AOS tender points (see below).

AOS TENDER POINTS
All patients were given a complete physical exam that emphasized the musculoskeletal system. During this exam, mild pressure was applied over the following areas (the AOS tender points) on both sides of the body:

- Lateral epicondyles (outer side of the elbow).
- Iliotibial bands (sides of the upper thigh).

- Gluteal/sciatic notch (middle/outer buttocks).
- Lumbar paraspinous (muscles on each side of the L3-through-L5 area of the lower spine).
- Upper trapezius (between the top of the shoulders and the neck).
- Lateral cervical/base of skull (where the back of the neck meets the skull).

The results of the exam were as follows: 100 percent of AOS patients had tenderness to at least one tender point; 78 percent had tenderness in two points; and 60 percent of AOS patients had tenderness in three or more points.

AOS TREATMENT
In an extensive history conducted of all patients, they related their chief complaint of pain, past medical history, history of previous surgeries and medications, family and social history, pain-prone personality style, current physical limitations and fears, spiritual history, and stressful events from their past and present circumstances.

After undergoing their physical exam (see above), they all attended two one-hour lectures explaining AOS—including its anatomy, physiology, and treatment. (The content of these lectures is presented in various ways throughout this book.) After the lectures, the patients were instructed to read AOS-related materials and do the homework I had assigned. Specifically, they were instructed to spend at least thirty minutes each day for four to six weeks on what in this book is called the Pain-Free for Life Program (outlined in chapter 8).

All patients were called between six and eight weeks and again six months after their office visit. They were asked, "How much improvement are you having in your pain: 0 to 20 percent, 20 to 40 percent, 40 to 60 percent, 60 to 80 percent, or 80 to 100 percent?"

After eight weeks, we were able to contact all fifty patients. After six months, we were able to reach forty-three patients. Here are the results:

🌿 AOS STUDY RESULTS		
	(50 PATIENTS)	**(43 PATIENTS)**
PAIN IMPROVEMENT	6- TO 8-WEEK RESULTS (% OF PATIENTS)	6-MONTH RESULTS
0–20% better	3 patients (6%)	2 patients (5%)
20–40% better	3 patients (6%)	2 patients (5%)
40–60% better	2 patients (4%)	1 patient (2%)
60–80% better	3 patients (6%)	3 patients (7%)
80–100% better	39 patients (78%)	35 patients (81%)

In other words, after only six to eight weeks, 78 percent of these AOS patients got 80 to 100 percent better. All were patients who had experienced chronic pain for an average of seven years, and who had "medical names" and "physical reasons" for their pain— or so they thought. The results continued and even improved at the six-month follow-up. Since that study, I've seen the same success over and over in my practice.

The Autonomic Overload Syndrome pain symptoms described in this chapter are extremely common. In fact, even if you don't have any AOS symptoms yourself, it's likely that someone in your family does. The negative effects of stress and repressed emotions are epidemic in our society today.

But now, even though you have a better understanding of how AOS manifests itself in your body, it's necessary to go a little deeper as we explore the scientific and biological causes of the syndrome. Then, you'll possess an even firmer understanding of the actual operation of AOS in your mind and body—and you'll be in a much stronger position to find ways to counter the painful effects of AOS in your own life.

WHAT'S REALLY CAUSING YOUR PAIN?

By now, you may suspect that you—or someone you know—has Autonomic Overload Syndrome. Also, you've seen the wide variety of symptoms this condition can produce. But most likely you are still wondering: *How exactly does AOS work to produce pain in my body? What is the science behind this syndrome?*

To answer these and related questions about the precise cause of your pain, let's reflect again on my working definition of AOS:

> *Autonomic Overload Syndrome (AOS) is a group of chronic pains and other symptoms caused by harmful levels of stress, pressure, and repressed strong negative emotions that have built up in the subconscious mind.*

As a preliminary step in examining this definition, we'll focus first on the meaning of *mind*—especially *subconscious mind*.

WHAT'S YOUR MIND ALL ABOUT?

There are many ways to understand how the mind may be related to the complexities of the human brain. But for the purposes of our AOS discussions, we'll think about the mind in just two ways: the *conscious* mind and the *subconscious* mind.*

You know a great deal about the conscious mind. It's the part of the brain that you use to say what you want to say, and do what you want to do—aiming and throwing a fishing lure just in front of the fish's mouth, for example, or deciding which big, juicy slice of pizza to buy. Generally speaking, your conscious mind thinks rationally (or *thinks* it does). With your conscious thoughts, you can cause yourself to give a speech, kick a ball, or clap your hands. Yet your conscious mind probably makes use of only about 10 percent of your brain—especially the frontal cortex. In contrast, most of your brain and bodily functions operate on a subconscious level.

WHEN YOUR SUBCONSCIOUS KICKS IN

Your subconscious mind, which operates just out of your sight and self-awareness, is involved in almost everything you do or think. The subconscious kicks in as you're driving your car—and you have to react without thinking if a child bolts out into the street in front of you. It's at work when you experience an unplanned daydream . . . or feel an urge to eat a tempting piece of chocolate . . . or sense your bowels squeezing in response to stress.

The subconscious mind is also involved in storing memories, generating dreams, and processing information, even when you're not consciously aware of that information. For example, we've all

---

*Although I believe that the mind and the brain are different entities, this distinction isn't important for understanding AOS—and I use the terms interchangeably. Also, for AOS purposes, I've found it helpful to refer to anything below the conscious level as simply *subconscious*.

made a so-called Freudian slip by saying something we didn't intend to say, often at an inappropriate moment. The slip is actually a subconscious thought spilling over into the conscious mind and through the lips—without any conscious act of the will.

For purposes of understanding AOS, it's helpful to think about two distinct functions of the subconscious mind:

- The subconscious participates in the activation and stimulation of the autonomic nervous system and what has popularly been called the stress response.
- The subconscious acts as a sort of storehouse or basement for all repressed emotions.

STRESS AND YOUR SUBCONSCIOUS

The science of AOS—and the causation of AOS pain—begins with stress, and with the emotions and physiological changes caused by stress. Although the term *stress* means different things to people, here is my working definition:

Stress is any threat to an individual's physical or psychological well-being, whether real, perceived, or imagined.

More than sixty-five years ago, Hans Selye recognized not only that stress protects the body, but also that too much stress can damage it. In the 1960s, University of Washington School of Medicine psychiatrists Holmes and Rahe found ways to quantify stressful events—and they concluded that too many stressful events in a short period of time is strongly associated with physical illness.

More recently, Bruce McEwen of the Rockefeller University has done extensive research on the physical and psychological effects of stress. McEwen uses the technical term *allostasis* to describe the ability of the body to maintain stability during stress and change. In a 2004 article published in the *Annals of the New York Academy of*

Sciences, McEwen describes the protective and damaging effects from stress: "When the [stress response] is not turned off after the stress is over . . . or when the [stress response] is overused by many stressors, there are cumulative changes that lead to a wear-and-tear called allostatic overload."[1]

In other words, short periods of stress—and the short bursts of the emotions produced by stress—are usually no problem. But as stress hormones and stress-related emotions build up day after day, the end result may be a cascade of problems for our mental and physical health—including AOS pain and symptoms.

PHYSICAL THREATS

Some types of stress can challenge or threaten our physical well-being. In days of old, the physical threats were easier to see: Vikings marching on the horizon, enemies throwing spears, or wild bears crashing through the woods. The physical threats needed a quick stress response, to make it easy to run as fast as possible and scream at the top of the lungs.

But in our contemporary society, threats to physical well-being are more subtle: The pressures of keeping a job, meeting the boss's deadlines, and making enough money all may appear to threaten our ability to feed and clothe ourselves and our families. And there always seem to be threats to physical health, whether from another terrorist attack or a heart attack.

All around us stress-producing messages say, *You'd better watch out or something may go terribly wrong!* So to defeat the terrorists, we all take off our shoes when we go through airport security. To avoid those cardiovascular threats, we adjust our consumption of carbs, or lose more weight.

PSYCHOLOGICAL THREATS

Most of the stresses we face as Americans, however, are threats to our psychological well-being—our sense of happiness or sense that things are going okay. There are many ways to describe this kind of stress: mental stress, work stress, financial stress, marriage stress, traffic stress, infertility stress, diet stress, political stress . . . the list goes on.

Realizing the American Dream by keeping up with the Joneses may be another source of continuous stress. Many of us constantly worry about buying the newest car, living in the right neighborhood, sending our kids to the best schools, or wearing the trendiest clothes. These anxieties seem to never stop—and in the end, they just wear us out.

In addition, we face constant stress trying to satisfy our own self-imposed psychological needs and demands. People who must be seen as nice and well liked all the time have the daily stress of making sure others are happy and think well of them. Every day their minds are stressed with the pressure of thoughts such as, *Oh no, maybe I said that wrong!* Or, *I think she's upset with me!* Or, *He must think I'm terrible—and I can't live with that.*

Other people may live and die by the respect or lack of respect they feel from others. These types are prone to constant stress that threatens their core desire to be held in high esteem. If you cut them off in traffic, interrupt them in the middle of a sentence, or forget to ask them to your party, they'll feel *dis*respected, and their stress response will stay on overdrive.

Still others may have a psychological need to be seen as competent, smart, and right all the time. The Perfectionist (see the following chapter), for example, experiences waves of daily stress trying to do everything on her list and always having to prove to herself and others that she's sharp—almost perfect. When things go wrong during the day, the Perfectionist's stress is real and almost palpable. Sometimes you can see the sweat beading on his forehead and the redness in his cheeks. But at other times, the Perfectionist will turn into what I call a professional emotion stuffer: You don't see any outward signs of anger—perhaps just a smile. Of course, what's going on *inside* is far from calm and can lead to all kinds of AOS symptoms.

REAL, PERCEIVED, OR IMAGINED THREATS

Stress can have the same effect on your body, whether it's real or imagined. So if you dream that you're a victim of armed robbery, your stress response will activate in the same way as if you actually *are* a victim of armed robbery. You've probably awakened from a terrible dream with sweat on your brow, your heart racing, and other signs of sheer panic. Even though you know it was all a dream, that won't matter; your mind and body have reacted to the stressful fear- and anxiety-producing dream as though the events in your sleeping mind were absolutely real.

In addition, the severity of a stress or threat is largely a matter of your overall perception of life. If you are basically a pessimist (the glass is always half empty, jobs are never done quite right), your life will tend to be more stress-filled than if you're an optimist (the glass is half full, jobs are usually done okay). In fact, if you're a pessimist, your overactivated stress response is very likely to have a negative impact on your health. According to a Mayo Clinic study, you have a *19 percent less chance of dying* if you're an optimist than if you're a pessimist.[2]

In another sense, you could say that stress really has no effect on you at all—that what really matters are the *emotions* caused by the stress in your life. In other words, it's not the bear, but the *fear* of the bear that sets off the stress response. If the bear were your pet, you wouldn't have a stress response at all. Likewise, it's not the gun that's stressful. Rather, it's the *anxiety* you may have that the gun will go off and kill you that sets off the stress response. It's not hearing, "Honey, my parents are coming to live with us" that's stressful. It's the *anger and anxiety* you feel that set off your stress response.

Understand that *stress results in strong emotions*, and the dangerous emotions drive the stress response. We'll talk more about these dangerous stress emotions a bit later. But now let's take a closer look at what happens inside your body when the stress produces strong emotions—in the form of what is known as the stress response.

How the Stress Response Works Inside You

Here's a diagram (figure A) to help guide you as we explore the stress response. The main message is that stress can result in strong emotions such as anger, fear, guilt, shame, and anxiety. Furthermore, these strong emotions activate the autonomic nervous system and lead to physical pain and related symptoms.

The major players in the stress response, which is also called the

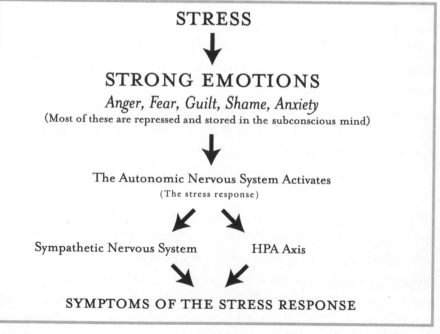

Figure A

fight-or-flight response, are the autonomic nervous system and the hypothalamic-pituitary-adrenal (HPA) axis. The subconscious mind (especially through the limbic system, or that part of the brain that I sometimes call the "emotional quarterback") helps influence many functions of the body—including the powerful autonomic nervous system. Also known as the automatic nervous system, the autonomic nervous system works without conscious thought. The autonomic system, which is part of the central nervous system, makes things happen in your body in one of two ways: by stimulating or by relaxing.

Furthermore, the autonomic nervous system consists of two parts: the sympathetic and the parasympathetic nervous systems. The sympathetic system, the more active of the two in the stress response, is activated through secretion of the powerful molecule adrenaline (also known as epinephrine). Both the sympathetic and parasympathetic systems can excite or relax different organs. In general, however, the sympathetic system stimulates or speeds up systems, organs, and body parts that help you run away from the bear if you have fear, or prepare you to fight the pickpocket thief when you're angry.

The problem arises when a stressful event causes a strong emotional response. For example, if a pickpocket has just stolen your wallet, you may explode in anger. That means your autonomic nervous system is turning on the adrenaline and causing the sympathetic system to increase your heart rate, pumping blood quickly to your muscles and brain. This response increases your blood pressure, metabolism, and muscle strength. At the same time, the autonomic nervous system opens up your lungs to receive more oxygen, releases sugar from the liver to feed the muscles, and activates the sweat glands to keep your internal engines cool as you tense your muscles to run after the thief. If you can imagine this pickpocket scenario, you can begin to experience how the stress response works.

But the autonomic nervous system is not the only biological mechanism that goes to work inside you in such situations. The autonomic system activates—or turns on to overdrive—its other partner in the stress response, the HPA axis, consisting of the hypothalamus, the pituitary gland, and the adrenal glands. Specifically, in response to the stress emotions, the hypothalamus portion of the brain sends signals to the pituitary gland. The pituitary then sends signals to the adrenal gland, and the adrenal gland pumps out lots of adrenaline (epinephrine), norepinephrine (noradrenaline), and cortisol into the bloodstream.

These stress-response molecules then begin to circulate in the blood, going to different organs to trigger important changes in the body: increasing blood sugar (to feed the muscles and brain), constricting the blood vessels, and dilating the pupils (to let more light into the eye).

Illustrations of the autonomic nervous system, figures B and C, should help you understand a little better what happens when you go on overdrive in your response to dangerous stress emotions.

THE AUTONOMIC "SPEEDOMETER"—A KEY TO AOS

As I mentioned briefly in chapter 1, one way to understand Autonomic Overload Syndrome is to think of the autonomic nervous system as a speedometer. First, let's say you're relaxed (see figure B), with your autonomic speedometer going at about thirty miles an hour. At this point, your lungs are open enough to breathe smoothly; your heart is beating about sixty-five times per minute; your muscle tone is relaxed, with no wads of painful muscle in your back; you're not sweating; the tiny blood vessels in your muscles are dilated, with oxygen-rich blood bathing the muscle fibers; your stomach is making just enough acid; your bowels are relaxed and moving unnoticeably smoothly; and your bladder is relaxed.

But now let's introduce a couple of strong emotions that will ac-

PAIN & SYMPTOMS

Conscious
Subconscious

Autonomic Nervous
System Relaxed

0   100

MUSCLES
The muscles are relaxed with good
blood flow.

HEART
The heart rate is normal
and even.

BRAIN
The autonomic systems sends
relaxed signals to the organs of
the body.

INTESTINES
The intestines squeeze
smoothly and unnoticeably.

Figure B

PAIN & SYMPTOMS

<u>Conscious</u>
Subconscious

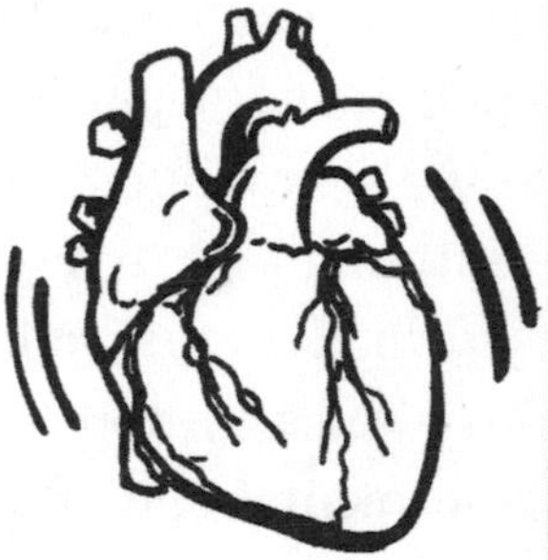

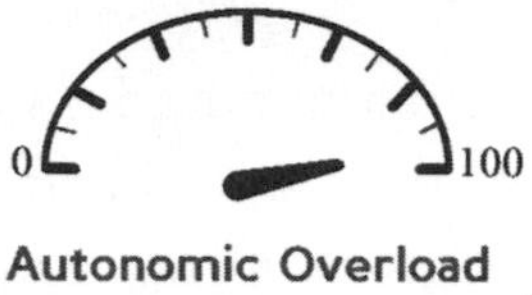

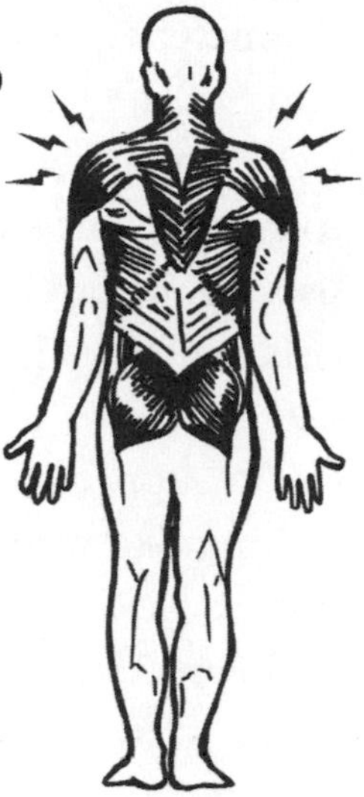

Autonomic Overload

0 _____ 100

MUSCLES
Muscle blood flow decreases and
muscle tone tightens, producing
muscle pain.

HEART
The heart rate increases.

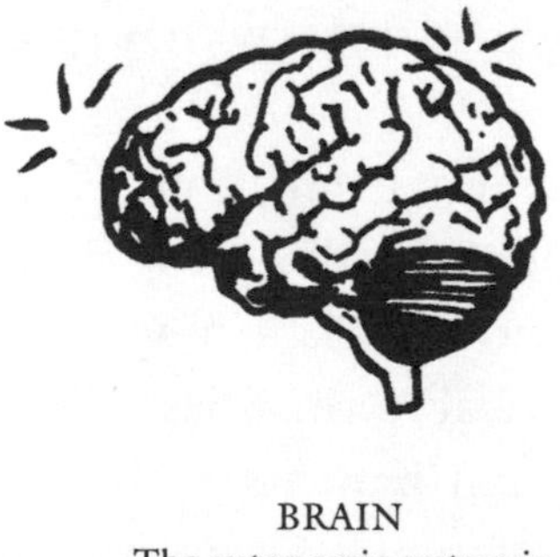

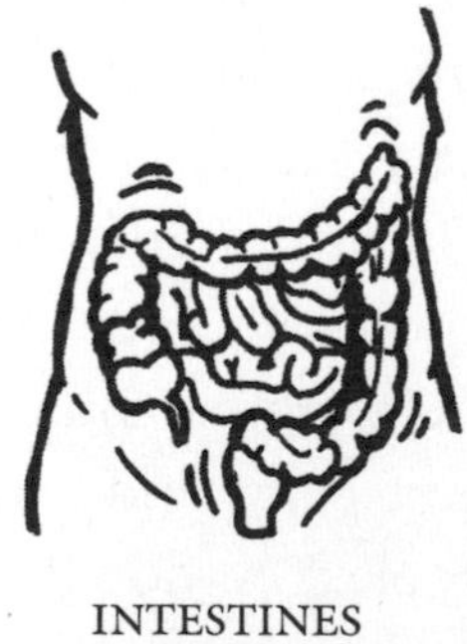

BRAIN
The autonomic system is
overloaded and sends *overdrive*
signals to the body.

INTESTINES
Stomach acid increases and
the bowels squeeze
tightly, producing
painful cramps.

Figure C

tivate the stress response. Suppose you're gripped by fear from an armed robbery, or by anger when your new car is struck from behind in an auto accident, or by sudden grief, fear, and loneliness after the death of someone in your family.

Now your autonomic speedometer turns up to a hundred miles an hour (see figure C). Your lungs dilate, and you begin to breathe faster. Your heart races, and your blood pressure increases. Your muscles tighten; you begin to sweat; your stomach makes a lot of acid, triggering heartburn. Also, your bowels cramp, you lose your appetite, and your blood vessels constrict (get tighter) in some areas to shunt blood to your brain.

Although the stress response is supposed to protect you, when it's turned on too high for too long—or when there aren't enough thirty-miles-an-hour downtimes between stressors—it begins to cause mental and physical problems. In effect, that's what happened with some individuals who were under significant stress in Baltimore a year or so ago.

DANGEROUS STRESS RESPONSES IN THE NEWS

Some in the media reacted with astonishment when a 2005 medical study in Baltimore reported that emotional stress had produced severe pain and heart problems in patients with no previous history of heart disease.

It all started when researchers from Johns Hopkins University School of Medicine concluded in the *New England Journal of Medicine* that anger, fear, or other disturbing emotions can cause chest pains and serious heart abnormalities in otherwise healthy people.[3] Although all nineteen patients in the study recovered, there was speculation that without the proper emergency treatment they received, they might have suffered debilitating injuries or even death.

The *New York Times* and other national news media immediately dramatized the report by styling these findings as examples of a "broken heart syndrome."[4] They noted that the victims, mostly women, had suffered heart problems as a result of high-stress emotions after such events as an armed robbery, a surprise party, an auto accident, and a death in the family.

As I reflected on this research, I remembered other studies that described the potentially devastating effects of an overloaded stress response—such as a *Lancet* article in September 1991, which reported the stress effects of the Scud missile attacks on Israel during the First Gulf War. Most of us recall that for several months, Iraq launched Scud missiles at Israel. Only one or two might hit each day, but this was enough to cause debilitating anger, fear, and even terror in Israeli citizens, who had no idea when they put their kids down to bed whether a missile would soon fall out of the sky and destroy their family.

The *Lancet* article referenced Israeli hospitals and physicians, who noticed dramatic and "sharp increases" in the incidence of acute myocardial infarction (MI, or heart attacks) and sudden death during these attacks. But the heart attacks weren't caused by the missiles; they were caused by the overloaded, always-turned-on stress response caused by continuous fear and anger.

Another article published by researchers Leor and Poole in the February 1996 *New England Journal of Medicine* pointed out that the emotional effects caused by the Los Angeles/Northridge earthquake served as triggers of sudden cardiac death.[5] In other words, the fear, panic, and anger associated with the earthquake caused autonomic overload, including constriction of the heart's blood vessels, among other problems. As a result, twenty-four people died of sudden cardiac death that day (the overall average was four deaths from sudden cardiac death per day).

More recently, researcher Sandro Galea published an article in the March 2002 *New England Journal of Medicine* discussing the aftermath of the September 11 terrorist attack in New York City.[6] The horrendous nature of the attack, with its loss of life and overwhelming stress, resulted in significant numbers of people suffering from depression, sleep disturbance, and chronic pain—all part of the condition known as post-traumatic stress disorder (PTSD).

Many times, when such stressful events and their accompanying emotions begin to wreak havoc inside the brain and body, pain symptoms emerge as part of the Autonomic Overload Syndrome.

LINKING THE STRESS RESPONSE TO YOUR AOS PAIN

As the speedometer regulating your autonomic nervous system revs up under stress, dangerous levels of stress-stimulated emotions overload the autonomic nervous system. In most cases, these emotions become firmly buried in the subconscious mind, thus causing the autonomic nervous system to remain constantly in the "on" position.

When autonomic overload occurs, pain and pain-related symptoms may appear, including the bowels squeezing and cramping with irritable bowel syndrome (IBS); peripheral blood vessels constricting and dilating to trigger migraine headaches; adrenaline levels rising to exacerbate insomnia; and stomach acid levels surging to produce heartburn.

In biological terms, here are some of the specific changes that occur in your body when your autonomic nervous system is overloaded and turned to the "on" position:

◆ Vasoconstriction (narrowing) of the tiny blood vessels (arterioles) within the muscles occurs. When the vessels are narrower, blood flow to the muscle is reduced, along with a reduction in the oxygen that the blood carries.
◆ The tone of the muscle changes, with contraction (tightening) of the muscle fibers occurring.
◆ Muscle nerve fibers (called C fibers), which are responsible for feeling pain, become more sensitive.

When it comes to muscle health—and a pain-free life—blood flow and oxygen are critical. I first learned in my gross anatomy class in med school that oxygen is necessary to relax a muscle. The reason a cadaver is so stiff and its muscles so tight is that there isn't any oxygen to relax the muscles.

Also, it takes blood flow to remove the pain-producing by-products of muscle use, such as lactic acid. Even a tiny reduction in blood flow may cause the muscle to cramp and become painful with lactic acid and C-fiber changes. This is why hot showers and massages tend to provide *short-term* relief of AOS muscle pain: They temporarily improve the blood flow and oxygen delivery to the painful muscles. But after the effects of the hot shower or massage wear off, AOS muscles return to their tight, painful, contracted state—because the autonomic speedometer is still turned up.

In clinical studies published in journals *Pain* and *Occupational Medicine*, Larsson and collaborators recorded levels of blood flow in the small-vessel circulation of people with chronic pain in the trapezius muscle (the muscle of the upper outer back and neck).[7] They found that blood flow was significantly lower on the more painful side of the body, and they also discovered an increase in muscle tension in those areas. In other words, due to autonomic sympathetic constriction of the tiny arterioles, the muscle that had chronic pain was not getting as much oxygen-rich blood. This reduced blood flow left those muscles more prone to pain, tightness, and spasms.

The *good news* with Autonomic Overload Syndrome is that your painful muscles are not facing any permanent damage. And the *great news* is that this pain-producing process can be stopped, because the autonomic nervous system can be turned down. In other words, with the proper mind–body–spirit treatment plan, it's really possible for you to become pain-free.

But in practical terms, how exactly can you manage the stress and stress-related emotions in your life better—and overcome your

AOS pain? The detailed answer to this question and description of specific treatments will come in chapter 8 and subsequent treatment chapters. But to begin preparing you to do battle with your pain, let's look a little more closely at the strategy used by your main opponent—your subconscious mind.

HOW YOUR SUBCONSCIOUS MIND HANDLES YOUR EMOTIONS

It would be easy to understand how your autonomic nervous system could become overloaded if Scud missiles were poised to hit your house every night, or if a bear chased you on the way to work every morning. But it's harder to understand how stress-related emotions are causing AOS pain symptoms when you feel calm on the outside and are living a life free of Scuds and bears.

The key to resolving this mystery—and understanding the link between AOS and your emotions—is this:

The dangerous emotions that cause Autonomic Overload Syndrome and chronic muscle pain are not *the ones that we see and feel, or that we're conscious of. Instead, the bad emotions are those we don't* see and feel because we've stuffed (repressed) them down *into the subconscious mind. As a result, these stress-stimulated emotions build up to dangerous levels in the subconscious mind, causing autonomic activation, pain, and AOS symptoms.*

In other words, instead of experiencing and constructively processing these dangerous emotions and feelings, our subconscious mind—and sometimes our conscious mind—sweeps them under the carpet. Also, the subconscious mind acts as the hard drive, storehouse, or basement—as I often put it—for all the memories and negative emotions we've repressed over the years. These repressed emotions build up over time, eventually overloading our autonomic nervous system. Repression is a powerful defense mechanism; it's a way we unconsciously cope with stressful emotions and the hard things about life.

THE ROOTS OF REPRESSION

Dr. John Sarno has said that for every "nickel of emotion" we consciously experience, we bury or repress "about ninety-five cents." Where do we stuff them? Answer: the subconscious mind.

Do we ever bury these strong negative emotions, thoughts, memories, and impulses consciously? Sometimes we do—and that's known as suppression.

For example, we may think, *I'm not going to think about that now. It's too much for me to handle.* So we consciously push the thought out of sight. In any case, whether we repress subconsciously or suppress consciously, the subconscious mind, or basement deep inside us, starts to fill up with strong negative emotions—and we begin to suffer from AOS.

Psychiatrist Sigmund Freud once summed up the repression issue this way as he was speaking to a packed auditorium:

> *Suppose that [in] this lecture room and among this audience, whose exemplary quiet and attentiveness I cannot commend enough, there is nevertheless someone who is causing a disturbance and whose poor mannered laughter, chattering and shuffling with his feet are distracting my attention from my task of lecturing. I have to announce that I cannot proceed with my lecture; and thereafter three or four of you who are strong men stand up, and after a short struggle, put the interrupter outside the door. So, now he is "repressed," and I can continue my lecture. But in order to keep the interrupter from entering the room once again and resuming his rude behavior, the strong men put my will into effect by placing their chairs up against the door as a*

*"resistance." If you will, now translate the two locations
concerned into . . . the conscious and unconscious, you will have
a fairly good picture of the process of repression.*[8]

A simplified AOS version of Freud's rather colorful illustration
might read something like this: Our conscious mind (or the subconscious mind itself) will push the rude emotion—the "interrupter"—out the door of consciousness into our subconscious
mind. The door leading back to the conscious mind is then locked.
But in the meantime, that rude emotion builds up in the subconscious through the process of repression. The end result is that the
buried emotion turns up the autonomic nervous system—and leads
to all sorts of health problems, including back pain, fibromyalgia,
and other AOS symptoms.

In any event, repression is our natural response to disturbing,
dangerous, and socially unacceptable emotions. It allows us to feel
a little emotion but not be overwhelmed by it. We may feel a bit of
irritation, but we can still keep a smile on our face, let it go, and
keep working. We may feel a little anxious, but we just get busy and
go on with our business; we don't become paralyzed with fear or
sidetracked by threatening emotions like anger.

I think a little of this repression is probably healthy. But most of
us are professional repressors. As already indicated, we probably repress 95 percent of our strong negative emotions, and most of the
time we're completely unaware of what's happening. These emotions are stored in our subconscious mind, where they build up
over time into a mountain of dangerous emotions causing continuous autonomic nervous system activation, muscle pain, and other
symptoms, as illustrated on p. 95.

When the dangerous emotions build up to a critical level like the
volcano in this picture (figure D)—or when, like the interrupter in
Freud's story, those emotions threaten to burst back into our conscious mind—the subconscious mind turns the autonomic nervous

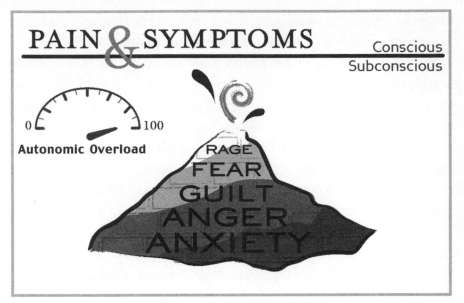

Figure D

system up to a hundred miles an hour or beyond, and we experience AOS pain symptoms.

Up to this point, I've made many references to negative emotions and suggested on a number of occasions what they may be. But now let's explore in more detail what the *most dangerous* emotions are—and how we can be sure that we'll recognize them.

THE MOST DANGEROUS EMOTIONS

Most of the time we don't repress happy emotions. When did you last decide to stuff happiness, or joyfulness, or hilarity? We usually like to express and savor these feelings. On the other hand, we do generally like to repress emotions that are dangerous or threatening in some way to our perceived identity or to our personal comfort.

We begin to repress strong negative emotions when we are small children because we don't want to become openly angry at our moms or dads: that could be dangerous to our well-being. Later on, we still don't want to acknowledge the extent of our strong

95

negative feelings toward people we respect because of a fear that they might lose respect for us or become angry with us.

In other words, the basic purpose of our repression is to support a defense mechanism that we think helps make us safe. The most dangerous emotions are the ones that could have the strongest negative impact on us socially and relationally. When repressed, these emotions also have the strongest impact on our autonomic nervous system and the pathways to AOS pain.

While this list is not exhaustive, the "trifecta" of the most dangerous emotions consists of anger, fear, and shame.

ANGER

The first and most dangerous emotion is anger. Like all emotions, anger isn't just an emotion; it is a "molecule of emotion," to paraphrase the title of the book by noted neuropeptide researcher Candace Pert. The anger molecule, whether expressed or repressed, produces enormous activation of our autonomic nervous system through the stress response. In fact, I've found that this buried emotion is the number one culprit in AOS pain.

Because most of us are reluctant to admit that we're angry, it's often helpful to start any exploration of our anger by looking at its less threatening cousins: frustration, irritation, and disappointment. These anger synonyms—as I like to call them—are generally much more palatable to my patients than anger itself. Most of us can't usually fathom that we're actually sitting on a mountain of *real* anger in our subconscious minds.

I can remember several female patients who couldn't think about anger, but they could talk about how "disappointed" they were with their friends or husbands. The typical male patient is more comfortable with the words *irritated* and *frustrated* when describing his spouse, co-worker, or boss. If I had to put anger on a scale of increasing severity, with each related word connoting a more dangerous set of feelings, the sequence would probably emerge this way: *bothered—disappointed—frustrated—irritated—ticked off—angry—enraged*.

In the end, though, it all comes down to a variation on the emotion of anger. We might feel or observe the anger emotion as it produces a red face, an increased heart rate, or—for those who are *really* angry—a loss of appetite. When the anger molecules build up over time into a mountain of dangerous emotion, the autonomic nervous system produces the symptoms you now understand to be AOS. (Remember, your autonomic system acts the same way whether the emotion arises from a concrete experience, a dream, or a repressed thought or memory.)

FEAR

The second powerful and extremely dangerous emotion that drives many AOS symptoms is fear. As with the other emotions, fear can assume many different faces. Adults, for instance, usually don't say they are afraid of something. Instead, they'll say: "I don't like that," or "I'm a little concerned about that," or "Let's not go there."

Related words, or fear synonyms that you might use to look for the repressed emotion of fear, include: *concerned—nervous—worried—anxious*. There are so many fears we experience: fear of the unknown, fear of death, fear of being out of control, fear of rejection, fear of being found out, fear of being alone, fear of being known, fear of being mediocre, fear of failure—to name just a few.

This emotion is a particularly important emotion for the People-Pleaser personality (see the following chapter). People-Pleasers fear that people won't think they're nice and won't like them. Since they are banking their identity on being perceived by others as good, nice people, it's a fearful prospect to risk upsetting others. Likewise, Perfectionists may also be plagued by stressful fears that crop up daily—fear of being average, fear of looking ridiculous, or fear of failing at a task. Different pain-prone personalities may fear different things.

Sometimes our repressed fears show up in our dreams. We may dream about what it would be like if our spouse divorced us, or if a loved one died, or if we lost our job. In fact, dreams may be one way that repressed fears are able to find a little release in ways other than pain.

But regardless of the form fear may take, repressed fear is a major driver of the autonomic nervous system and facilitator of AOS.

SHAME

The next most powerful autonomic-overloading emotion—the very dangerous emotion of shame—is sometimes quite hard to pull to the surface.

For example, when many of my patients in the depth-journaling phase of their treatment (see chapter 9) are looking for their repressed, subconscious shame, they don't get very far, at least not at first. Instead, they move around the issue by focusing on the "embarrassment that made me feel small," or the "comment that embarrassed me," or "the person who belittled me." The term *humiliated* is another common synonym for shame. If I ranked the related words for shame, the list would read something like this: *embarrassed—guilty—humiliated—disgraced—shame.*

A close cousin, and in many ways a subcategory, of shame is *guilt.* If we are ashamed of the way we have acted, we often feel guilty about it. With some people, guilt can get out of control or become unmanageable.

For example, a Perfectionist may set impossibly high standards of conduct for herself, and then become ashamed or feel guilty because she fails to live up to the ideal. I recall one female AOS back pain patient who had set a series of unreachable goals for herself as a working mother. She wanted to reach the top management level in her company *and* go to every one of her children's after-school functions *and* cook every evening meal at home. She was guilt-ridden about her inability to be a good mother and provide for her family—and as a result, she felt deep shame.

Another common cause of deep repressed shame is sexual abuse. The numbers are staggering: So many children and young adults are sexually abused. And as if the abuse alone weren't evil enough, these victims often feel a deep and lifelong sense of shame—as though they had something to do with provoking the abuse.

I've found that even if you've thought about an abuse and tried to get over it, you've probably just scratched the surface. There's likely a mountain of repressed shame associated with the event that has been too painful to process. But unprocessed and repressed shame will continue to activate and overload our autonomic nervous system—and many times the result will be physical pain and other AOS symptoms.

So what does all this have to do with your pain?

Just this: The AOS pains that may be plaguing you right now are the result of a buildup of strong, negative, repressed emotions. Most likely, when you begin to experience anxiety, fear, or anger from excessive stress and pressure, you don't deal with those emotions effectively. You are probably acutely aware that expressing these dangerous emotions openly is not socially acceptable or even safe for maintaining good relationships. So instead of expressing them, you slip into the habit of regularly *burying*, or repressing, these emotions without even thinking about it. As a result, your autonomic nervous system becomes excessively activated and overloaded. The end result is constricted micro blood vessels, tight and oxygen-deprived muscles, and various pains and other symptoms throughout the body.

A large component of the Pain-Free for Life Program involves uncovering the pain-producing mountain of repressed emotions and understanding where these emotions come from. At the same time, many of us have certain embedded personality traits that make us more susceptible to chronic pain than others. In fact, as we'll see in the next chapter, one of the biggest culprits in producing and magnifying large amounts of strong negative emotions inside us each day—and triggering AOS pain—is our particular pain-prone personality.

UNDERSTANDING YOUR PAIN-PRONE PERSONALITY

Erin was named Teacher of the Year three years in a row—the second-grade teacher whom all the parents of first-graders were vying for. Moms and dads knew that Erin was naturally sweet and kind, but she was also ultra-organized and had a way of getting things done. Her classes were well disciplined and orderly; every school day had a theme, and every theme had four or five fun activities to help the kids learn.

Though consistently punctual and efficient, she was always smiling and nice—never showing any signs of irritation. Erin held to a strong belief that learning could happen best when the day was well planned out and the kids were loved. But at the age of thirty, she realized that her teaching career was about to come to an end because of chronic back and neck pain.

Erin had been in continuous pain for seven years. Her symptoms began in her midtwenties with pain to her shoulder and neck muscles, including a muscle tightness and sometimes a burning sensation. The pain eventually spread to her midback, and she sometimes felt pain on the side of her elbow. All these pains increased to the point that she suffered almost every minute of the day. In addition, she had virtually no energy, making the task of getting through a full day with second-graders almost impossible. Then came the headaches and jaw pain. Her doctors told her that she had several problems: fibromyalgia, migraine headaches, tennis elbow, and TMJ syndrome (pain in the jaw, or temporomandibular joint).

After Erin had endured years of suffering, a friend—who had suffered similar symptoms but now was pain-free—told her one day about the Brady Institute for Health. I spent about an hour with Erin, exploring her medical history, her list of medications and previous diagnoses, her psychological history, her spiritual history, and finally her lab work, X-rays, and physical exam. She represented a classic case of Autonomic Overload Syndrome, which manifested itself as fibromyalgia, with such symptoms as fatigue, muscle aches, headaches, and irritable bowel. She also had AOS symptoms of epicondylitis (tennis elbow) and jaw pain in the temporomandibular joint.

We reviewed the list of dangerous repressed emotions that were overstimulating her autonomic nervous system and causing her pain. Next, we explored what could have caused the enormous mountain of dangerous emotions in the first place.

Her past was punctuated by many significant stresses and dangerous emotions. Her present circumstances were filled with the usual, sometimes overwhelming stresses associated with being a wife, mother, and teacher. But while she was describing her life, I noticed that she used phrases like *time management* and *can't do it right* to describe the frustration of her daily routine. She also said such things as, "You must think I'm terrible," and "They'll be so upset with me," and "I know I shouldn't think that way." These phrases were dead giveaways for the biggest cause of repressed and dangerous emotions in her subconscious mind: her *pain-prone personality.*

Erin fit into two pain-prone personality types: the Perfectionist and the People-Pleaser. Together, these tendencies caused her huge amounts of dangerous emotions on a daily basis, which had built up in her subconscious mind and resulted in her chronic AOS pain.

You've already been introduced to several of these pain-prone personality types through various case illustrations. For example, you know from chapter 1 that Susan was a Perfectionist. Here, you see that Erin is both a People-Pleaser and Perfectionist—a classic double-whammy pain combination—just like me (see chapter 2).

In fact, in my clinical experience with AOS patients, I have identified five major kinds of pain-prone personalities. These are categories of personal features and attitudes that make people more inclined to build up toxic levels of dangerous repressed emotions in their subconscious minds. The five are:

1. The Perfectionist.
2. The People-Pleaser.
3. The Legalist.
4. The Stoic.
5. The Fear-Prone.

As you learn about these personalities, remember that the main question to keep in mind is this: *How does my particular personality cause dangerous emotions—and therefore predispose me to AOS pain?* Also, remember that your personality will stay with you for life, but *you don't have to become a victim of pain*—not if you're aware of the dangerous emotions often associated with your personality, and if you make a commitment to avoid repressing those emotions.

Now let's take a closer look at the various pain personalities— and see where you might fit in.

THE PERFECTIONIST PERSONALITY

If you're a Perfectionist, you are conscientious, productive, and achievement-oriented. Being an extremely careful person, you like all tasks and projects to be completed to the final detail, without any flaws. Everything needs to be done right, and you have a clear understanding of what that means, from the correct way to wash the car to the right way to iron a shirt or fit dishes into the dishwasher.

Perfectionists are good organizers; they enjoy things being neat and tidy. They also like control, correctness, and orderliness. Perfectionists aren't perfect, but they'd like to be. If you're a Perfectionist, you tend to be a driven person, highly motivated, and self-critical.

On the positive side, you're probably quite responsible and dependable in your work and activities. But you consistently set long lists of impossible standards and goals for yourself and others. And if you finally get to the point that you accomplish your list, you allow yourself only a brief period to relax—because tomorrow you'll think of other things you need to do.

I tell my patients, "If a Perfectionist wins the Nobel Peace Prize, his acceptance speech would go something like this: 'Thank you, thank you, I appreciate this prize, but I think I could have done it better—and I probably should have done it much sooner.'" Instead of relieving the pressure, prizes and accolades often do the opposite—they put more pressure on the Perfectionist to do it again next year.

Perfectionists don't like being wrong or corrected; it goes against their deep need to be *right*. When you're a Perfectionist, a task or job is usually an all-or-nothing affair: It's either done right, or it's done wrong. The words *mediocre* and *not bad* make your stomach curdle.

Although most of your personality is something you're born with, a Perfectionist personality grows and thrives as you constantly try to prove to yourself and others that you're not inadequate or average. As competent as you may seem on the outside, you're driven internally by an inner fear of inadequacy and a need to *prove yourself* by achieving.

For the Perfectionist, life is filled with pressure—most of which is self-imposed. Of course, no one can achieve such high standards with no mistakes. And when you do slip up or fail to complete your tasks the right way—or when others don't complete their tasks the way you want, you're flooded with waves of strong negative emotion. As you or others around you fall short of your goals and lists, irritation, frustration, and anger are typical emotions that you, as a Perfectionist personality, face every hour of the day. In addition, the Perfectionist may experience a strong sense of guilt, feelings of inadequacy, and sometimes a fear of being found out to be far less than perfect—or possibly even average.

In the end, you regularly bury (repress) strong negative emotions, such as anger, deep in your subconscious because expressing such raw, unpleasant emotions isn't socially acceptable; it just isn't the right thing to do. But the reservoirs of repressed, toxic emotions continue to grow because you and those around you can never realize your impossible performance expectations.

Ironically, though, if you or a loved one or a colleague should happen to actually meet one of your goals, you won't celebrate the success or even dwell on it with satisfaction for more than a few moments. Self-congratulation is not acceptable for a Perfectionist. Instead, fearful of becoming complacent, you quickly move on, setting even higher goals to achieve tomorrow.

All in all, you live by a special credo, which could be stated this way:

THE PERFECTIONIST'S MOTTO

I must be perfect and right . . . I refuse to be average.

Others should watch what I do and say—and then follow my lead.

There are two ways of doing things in life: my way and the wrong way.

If I do fail, I'll just try harder . . . I hate it when I make mistakes.

I cover up my faults, my failures, and my inadequacies.

Life is hard, my lists are long, and I live with constant pressure.

Life is most fun when I can get everything done—the *right* way.

I get angry a lot with others, irritated by their incompetence and their laziness, but the one who frustrates and disappoints me the most . . . is *me*.

If you feel that the above profile and the accompanying mottoes describe you fairly well, you're probably a Perfectionist personality. Although it's very common for people with this personality to develop symptoms from Autonomic Overload Syndrome, remember that your pain-prone personality doesn't need to change for you to recover from AOS. You merely have to recognize the dangerous emotions you've been repressing due to your personality tendencies.

If you think you may be a Perfectionist, get out some paper and try this preliminary exercise. Answering these questions will help you begin to see yourself better, giving you a head start with your Pain-Free for Life Program.

Preliminary Questions to Unmask Your Perfectionist Personality

- Make a list of three things you didn't do right in the past week.
- What expectations do you put on yourself? List as many as you can.
- What are your expectations of others? Again, list as many as you can.
- What three things frustrate you most about yourself or others?
- What specific pressures did you put on yourself this week?
- How do you feel when you don't do something well?
- How do people make you angry most often?

THE PEOPLE-PLEASER PERSONALITY

While the drive of the Perfectionist is to be right, the drive of the People-Pleaser is to be accepted or well liked. People-Pleasers are nice and kind and sensitive people. They care deeply about what others think of them, and are always worrying if they may have angered or disappointed someone, or how someone else might feel about them.

If you're a People-Pleaser personality, you are generally other-centered or other-directed. In other words, you tend to put others before yourself because it's the good and nice thing to do, even when you don't want to be so generous. You rarely interrupt others or make abrupt and hasty decisions.

Another stress in the life of a People-Pleaser is relational conflict. To avoid conflict, you rarely tell other people what you really think of them. And although you may have strong opinions, you usually won't strongly disagree with anyone openly. Your careful avoidance of stressful relational situations is fueled by a deep inner fear of inadequacy and a fear that you won't be accepted by others, though you're probably not fully aware of these feelings. On the whole, most people would describe you as a happy, sweet, and nonconfrontational person.

As a People-Pleaser, you may also be involved in constantly rearranging your own plans—and neglecting your personal desires—to meet the wishes of others in an attempt to make them happy. You want to avoid potential conflicts, and you try hard not to hurt anyone else's feelings. As a result, you may often fail to tell the whole truth about a situation when you're conversing with people you care about. Chances are you're also a chronic peace negotiator, trying to make everyone feel good about everyone else when stressful situations arise.

People-Pleasers are usually giving, warm, kind, and empathetic people. If you're the kind of person that bakes cookies for the new neighbors even though you're busy and have lots of other things to do, you're probably a People-Pleaser. If you're crushed by someone being disappointed in you, you're probably a People-Pleaser.

The truth is, you were born with a nice and sweet way about you. But as you grew up, you developed a deep *need* to be good in the eyes of others and to be liked by everyone. To this end, you're always quite helpful to others, and always ready to sacrifice your needs for theirs.

People-Pleasers are wonderful people; however, they aren't as wonderful and nice as they'd like others to believe. No one is! Neglecting your own personal desires and needs while pasting a smile on your face can cause frustration, irritation, and even anger. As a result, this personality engages in a lot of cover-up. The word *anger* will seem quite foreign to you; you probably prefer to use the term *disappointed*.

Nevertheless, it takes a lot of energy and planning to be nice all the time, and this effort can be frustrating. So you have to be careful to cover up (or repress) those ugly thoughts or responses that are always threatening to break out. Also, all relationships in some way involve conflict, stress, and disappointment. To mask any negative responses to such difficulties, you have to be alert all the time. All this internal effort and repression sets you up to suffer from AOS pain.

The People-Pleaser's motto might read something like this:

THE PEOPLE-PLEASER'S MOTTO

I must be good, and nice . . . I'm not a bad or selfish person.
I will be happy, pleasant, and liked by everyone.
Whatever you do, please don't reject me.
I will put others before myself, because that's the good thing to do.
Of course, it takes a lot of energy to smile and be nice all the time, but I can usually swallow any anger and or bad thoughts I have.
Close relationships are hard for me—because I hate conflict.
If I told people what I really think, they'd be shocked!
I sometimes feel guilty, because I know I'm not as nice as people think I am . . . but because I work hard at it, I know I'm *not bad*!

If you feel that the above profile and the accompanying motto describe you fairly well, you're probably a People-Pleaser personality. To understand your personality type better—and to fathom the waves of dangerous emotions it causes you to repress—try this exercise. As with the Perfectionist, answering these questions will give you a head start with your Pain-Free for Life Program in part 2.

Preliminary Questions to Unmask Your
People-Pleaser Personality

- Do you constantly try to reduce relational conflict? Explain.
- Are you really as nice and sweet as you lead others to believe?
- What disappoints you? Describe how it feels.
- What do you think would happen if you told everyone what you really think about them? Be specific.
- How do you sacrifice your own needs for those of others?
- How do you feel when you sense others don't like you or are disappointed with you?
- What things make you feel guilty?

THE LEGALIST PERSONALITY

The dominant theme of the Legalist is this: "I'm okay because I do what's right and I keep my commitments."

The Legalist personality is similar in some ways to the Perfectionist: The Perfectionist likes to *do* things right but the Legalist likes to *be* right in almost every situation or topic of discussion. When a Legalist makes up her mind about something, she commits wholeheartedly to it and rarely changes her mind.

The Legalist is characterized by considerable rigidity and dogmatism in personal beliefs, values, and worldview. Those beliefs may be rooted in a particular religious commitment; in strong political convictions; or in a cause. Those who are fervent activists for First Amendment rights, women's rights, environmentalism, or any other personal philosophy may fit into this category. Legalists can be either conservative or liberal in their political or religious views, but a common trait is that they will argue their point of view as long and hard and passionately as anyone possibly can.

Legalists are both responsible and sensible. They're strongly committed to keeping their word. For this reason, they often take time before making big commitments and promises. Legalists are careful and deliberate when approaching a potentially close relationship—they may evaluate a potential partner by making lists and checking things off like a report card.

For many Legalists, life has to make sense and must preserve the heritage and commitments of the past. Some Legalist men, for example, may *demand* a traditional household structure, where the male works and his wife stays at home. They won't settle for anything else. The Legalist female may hold to rigid convictions about the right way to raise her children, and be unwilling to accept any advice that's even slightly different from her position.

On the whole, Legalists honor their commitments and expect others to honor theirs as well. Legalists tend to pay a great deal of attention to details and to following the rules in different social and business situations. As a result, they may be quick to find fault with others. To correct these faults, Legalists like to give lots of "constructive criticism." Because of their strong belief that *they are right*, Legalists are often very judgmental and display a critical attitude and intolerance toward others who don't hold to their same beliefs.

But here's a caveat: Passion and exclusivity in personal beliefs do *not* mean that you are definitely a Legalist. In other words, you may believe that your religious faith or political cause or personal worldview is the only logical, right, and true way to believe. But that doesn't automatically mean you are a Legalist who has trouble interacting with or accepting or learning from those of a quite different viewpoint.

The history of great religious and political movements is populated with those who hold strong beliefs—and often automatically find themselves in disagreement with those whose beliefs are different. Again, such strong personal convictions don't necessarily translate into intolerance or an inability to work with others. For example, Jesus was as exclusive about his beliefs as anyone could be—to the point that he was even willing to die for those beliefs. But he was inclusive in his expressions of love and compassion for others who didn't share his beliefs. This approach is different from that often taken by Legalists, who don't display much love for people they regard as wrong and who tend to dislike being around people who disagree with them.

Many Legalists judge themselves by the same tough standards that they apply to others, and therefore, Legalists often don't love themselves very well. They carry around a deep-seated sense of unworthiness and feel that they must earn the love of others (and God). Sometimes filled with self-contempt, they may believe that they don't really deserve to be loved. Instead, they are more comfortable trying to *earn* the love of others (even God). But on their own personal worthiness scale, they most likely rank themselves ahead of almost everyone they know.

Because of their inherent rigidity, Legalist personalities are highly susceptible to irritation and anger. But as with the other pain-prone personalities, irritation and anger in the Legalist are emotions that are usually stuffed and repressed rather than expressed.

Also, Legalists experience a lot of personal guilt and hidden fear. The guilt is related to knowing or suspecting that they're not really being as right as they think they are—or should be. The fear (and often anxiety) is related to being found out by others. As with the other pain-prone personalities, the Legalist's growing storehouse of toxic repressed emotions often emerges in the form of various aches and pains related to Autonomic Overload Syndrome.

Here's the motto I've written to help describe the life of a Legalist. As you look it over, remember that even though this motto may reflect your pain-prone personality, your personality can be overcome with the Pain-Free for Life Program.

THE LEGALIST'S MOTTO

I enjoy being right in almost every discussion and conversation.

I think my beliefs are right for me *and* right for everyone.

I'm nice to people, but I still feel like they're wrong a lot.

Most people in the world need to rethink their views.

Our culture would be better off if everyone did what I do.

Accepting unconditional love is hard for me.

Sometimes I fume after a particularly bad argument.

It's hard for me to be around people who are really different from me, but I can usually swallow any anger and keep things under control.

Most of my friends agree with most of my beliefs and positions.

God seems a bit impersonal to me—but he's always right and I try to be.

People think I criticize them a lot, but I'm just trying to help.

If you feel the above profile and the accompanying motto describe you fairly well, you're probably a Legalist personality. Here are a few questions for you to think about and answer if you're concerned that you might fit into this category. As with the other pain-prone personality types, answering these questions will give you a head start with your Pain-Free for Life Program in part 2.

Preliminary Questions to Unmask Your Legalist Personality

- What personal beliefs or views do you hold that you have trouble discussing with others? Give specifics.

- Do you get into arguments that have something to do with your strongly held convictions? Explain.
- Describe your last friend who disagreed with you a lot. What happened?
- Do you become angry easily when you discuss your beliefs with others who disagree with you?
- Do you find yourself friend-hopping and church-hopping because you end up disagreeing about something important?
- How do you feel when you sense others don't agree with you? Describe your thoughts and emotions in detail.
- What makes you the most angry?

THE STOIC PERSONALITY

Steven and Deborah had just driven about four hours for an evaluation of his chronic back pain. When I called Steven back to my office, his wife insisted that she come along: "I know he won't tell you everything, Dr. Brady," she explained. "So I need to be there."

Both were in their early seventies, and Steven was a successful businessman. His wife helped keep the books for the business.

As the exam progressed, Steven answered all my questions nicely and politely. He was a matter-of-fact kind of guy. When we got to the part of the exam where I take a psychological and spiritual history, he had even less to say. The questions seemed to bother him a little—as though I were being too personal. I don't think he was intentionally trying to avoid opening up about himself; the process of revealing more just seemed to strike him as unnatural, uncomfortable, and awkward.

Then Deborah piped up: "You see, Dr. Brady, he won't say anything. He's always been like this. He's almost always calm, and he never gets angry out loud or anything. But I know when he's upset because he disappears from the house and goes into his garage for a couple of hours."

Steven's behavior and his wife's descriptions of him helped me label him as a classic Stoic personality—a pain personality type that had contributed to the chronic back condition he had struggled with for years. With his type identified, we were in a position to move forward with the most effective treatment plan.

Stoicism, by the way, was one of the philosophical movements of the ancient Hellenistic period. The Stoics believed that strong emotions such as fear or envy or passionate love were weak and childish, and were to be avoided. They thought that smart sage-like people who attained high moral and intellectual levels would not have (or at least would not *show*) these strong emotions. Although the philosophy of classic Stoicism is now ancient history, the general personality characteristics of the Stoic are still around—and people with this personality type are pain-prone, with a tendency to produce symptoms of AOS.

So what are some of the common traits of the pain-prone Stoic?

Stoics are uncomfortable with having or expressing strong emotions—anger, abounding joy, passionate love, or deep sorrow. To the Stoic, a sense of strength comes from having emotions under control; the emotionless state feels powerful and stable. If you're a Stoic, you probably don't *intend* to repress strong emotions; you've just reached the point where you don't *feel* many strong emotions.

The Stoic personality is frequently found in men ages fifty and older, who think it's manly to keep a stiff upper lip in emotional situations. Crying at the movies, in a religious service, or at a funeral is way out of bounds. When the Stoic does cry, he often feels weak or senses he has acted inappropriately.

There are also a substantial number of women in this personality category. Some older women have been taught that the expression of emotions in public is not appropriate or classy. Younger women, especially those on a high-powered career track, may become more Stoic after they decide they can't express emotions at the office—

because that will interfere with their ability to advance in the corporate system. The underlying assumption is that a teary-eyed woman executive "just isn't management material."

Unfortunately, this radical avoidance of emotional expression unintentionally makes Stoics master repressors. In order to maintain balance and feel comfortable, Stoics often deny that they experience many strong emotions. Stoics might acknowledge feeling a *little* angry or guilty or even fearful, but their face doesn't show it because they allow themselves to experience only a small fraction of the emotion while subconsciously repressing almost all of it.

The result of Stoics' commitment to avoid strong emotions is a regular subconscious buildup of the very emotions they're trying to avoid. On a daily basis, their personality combines with the circumstances of life to cause an almost continuous repression of irritation, anger, frustration, shame, fear, and guilt.

The world of the Stoic may appear to her to be under complete control—until she wakes up one morning and, after she picks up her briefcase, her back "grabs." Months later, the back continues to hurt, despite multiple structural diagnoses and treatment prescriptions by well-meaning medical people. Now, the Stoic is racked with chronic back pain or some other symptom of AOS—as was the case with Steven in the illustration above.

If you are a Stoic and you were asked to affirm a particular credo or motto, what would it be? Consider this:

THE STOIC'S MOTTO

I'm uncomfortable with strong emotions—I've always been this way.
I don't cry much; it doesn't get you anywhere and seems so out of control.

I'm not *trying* to hide my emotions; it's just that I don't feel
the way others do.

If I bottle up my emotions effectively, I'll avoid all sorts of
problems.

If I can just put a cap on my emotions, I will be perceived
as strong.

I admire people who are strong and seem to be in control.

If I know a situation is likely to arise that will make me
openly emotional, I'll just avoid that situation.

If I showed people how I really feel, they'd be shocked!

A stiff upper lip is always preferable to a teary eye.

If you feel the above profile and the accompanying motto describe you fairly well, you're probably a Stoic personality. In my experience, these types rarely admit that they're Stoics, so it's often
helpful to ask your spouse or close friend if you might be one. To
understand this personality better, try answering these questions. As
with the other pain personalities, answering these questions will give
you a head start with your Pain-Free for Life Program in part 2.

Preliminary Questions to Unmask Your Stoic Personality

- On a scale of one to ten, with one being unrestrained and ten
  being very restrained, how restrained are you about showing
  your emotions?
- What's the most traumatic event that ever happened to you?
  How did you handle your emotions at that time?
- When you did express strong emotions in the past, what did
  it feel like?
- Are you embarrassed about crying in front of your spouse?
  Your best friend?

- Do you feel anxious when you're in an emotional situation?
- How do you express your anger?
- Do most people around you even know when you're angry?

THE FEAR-PRONE PERSONALITY

You may be a Fear-Prone pain personality if you are always antici-pating that the worst will happen . . . or if you think you're weak and frail . . . or if you feel that life in general is stacked against you. Consider the situation faced by one of my patients, Hannah.

The wife and mother of three children, Hannah suffered from chronic neck and upper back pain for nearly a decade. X-rays of her spine revealed degenerative disk disease, but nothing needing surgery. Her neck was tight, with wads of tender muscles through-out. In addition to the muscle pain, she often suffered with bouts of stomach cramps and diarrhea—diagnosed as irritable bowel syn-drome.

After taking a complete medical history and finishing the physi-cal exam, I asked Hannah about her life and about the biggest stresses in her day. Without hesitation, she said, "I'm afraid that one of my kids will die."

She continued: "It doesn't just stop there. I know it's unreason-able, but I'm always thinking about how I'm going to have to cope with life once something bad happens. It never does, but just the fear of it can give me anxiety—and diarrhea. It's my natural re-sponse to be fearful. I fear my husband dying, and I think of how my daughters and I can cope without him and how I would handle my kids' sadness. My mind thinks of scenarios that most likely will never, ever happen, but that is my immediate response. Last night I looked in the bedroom for one of my kids, but she wasn't there. I immediately thought someone had probably come into the house and abducted her. But she was actually just in the next room. For me, there seems to be *always* something to be fearful about—my mind just jumps from one thing to another. When I have a stomach pain, I think I might have ovarian cancer. I feel so much pressure trying to figure out how I can keep my kids safe."

I determined that Hannah's pain came from Autonomic Overload Syndrome. Her Fear-Prone personality had created *tons* of continuous pressure and anxiety and fear—which had resulted in dangerous repressed emotions. On the physical level, her autonomic overactivation had caused her to experience chronic neck and upper back muscle tightness, along with irritable bowel syndrome.

In my practice, people with severe fibromyalgia symptoms frequently have a bit of the Fear-Prone personality that plagued Hannah. But Fear-Prone people can present very different faces—from the socially outgoing to the quiet and withdrawn. The outgoing types may form relationships, even making an effort to meet new people. However, these particular Fear-Prone people tend to keep their acquaintances at a distance. In other words, outgoing Fear-Prone people actually avoid *intimacy* rather than people, and are fearful of what others think of them (in a way similar to the People-Pleaser personality).

Withdrawn Fear-Prone people project a different look, characterized by timidity and withdrawal. They may also mistrust most people for quite a while until they start to feel safer and more comfortable around them. Fear-Prone people often test others to determine whether or not they're being sincere in their friendliness. For that reason, their almost constant wariness of people makes them appear shy and sometimes aloof.

Withdrawn Fear-Prone people may use their shyness as a way to prevent others from becoming close, hurting them in the process. They may also feel and see rejection where it does not exist. In many cases, they have difficulty beginning and maintaining relationships, partly because they have difficulty trusting others.

People with a Fear-Prone personality tend to feel that life is out of control. They think a lot about the worst possibilities of any situation. If it's storming, they're thinking about tornadoes; if their child is out of sight for a second, their mind goes straight to thoughts of kidnapping or death. They *expect* loss or harm. In a rather strange twist, they may feel that their mental anticipation of danger can somehow prevent the danger from ever happening.

The Fear-Prone personality is easily scared by physicians. "It's just an innocent lump" sounds like "It's cancer." Or "You have fibromyalgia" sounds like "You have something mysterious, abnormal—and probably deadly—in your body."

The dominant emotions felt (and buried) by those in this category are fear and anger. From the above description of their traits, it's easy to understand why they think they have a lot to fear. But underneath that fear is an ocean of anger—because life is dangerous and out of control, people are hurtful, nature is unpredictable, and their bodies may have mysterious abnormalities.

Fear-Prone people usually don't see themselves as being angry because the anger is covered over by the obvious surface emotions: fear and worry. But like many pain-prone personalities, anger seems often to be the main culprit driving the overloaded autonomic nervous system to produce a variety of AOS symptoms.

Here's a sample Fear-Prone personality motto. Perhaps it describes a small part or the predominant part of your personality.

THE FEAR-PRONE'S MOTTO

It's hard not to think about dangerous and scary things.
Life seems totally out of control; nothing is certain anymore.
I don't think a day passes without my being worried about
    something.
I'm afraid to push myself physically; it might be too much
    for me.

I'm afraid that I've got something wrong with my body—
     something that no one can figure out.
It takes a lot of energy to have so much anxiety and fear—
     yet not make it obvious to everyone else what I'm think-
     ing about.
I can usually hide my fears and any anger or resentment I
     have. But sometimes, when things build up, I break down.
If I told people everything I really think, they'd think I'm
     nuts, and maybe the weakest person alive!
Thinking about the unknown makes me feel uptight.

If you feel the above profile and the accompanying motto describe you fairly well, you're probably a Fear-Prone personality. To
understand this personality type better, try responding to these
questions.

Preliminary Questions to Unmask Your
Fear-Prone Personality

* How many things can you think of right now that you're
  worried about? List them.
* Is it hard for you to really trust others in relationships?
* Do you become frustrated or even angry because you sense
  the constant threat of danger?
* What are the main pressures you feel in life? List them in
  detail.
* In life, do you usually go for it, or do you more often
  approach things with caution?
* Do you commonly expect bad things to happen?
* What is your greatest fear in life?

THE COMBO PERSONALITY

About two-thirds of my AOS patients seem to identify with one of the above five major pain-prone personalities. The other third are a *mixture* of pain-prone personalities—usually two of them. As a result, I often refer to them as Combo personalities.

As I've said, I'm both a Perfectionist and a People-Pleaser—and so is Erin, whose story is told at the beginning of this chapter. And by the way, this particular Combo personality is very common. I like to call it the double whammy, because if you're not facing irritation and anger from your Perfectionist side, you certainly are from the People-Pleaser side.

Also, *in general*, the more severe and pervasive your pains, the more likely it is that you have more than one set of pain personality traits. For this reason, Combo pain personalities typically suffer from the more complex chronic pain packages, such as fibromyalgia (though, of course, this isn't always the case).

Is it harder to be cured of your AOS pain if you incorporate more than one pain personality type? Definitely not! If you do have a combination of pain-prone personality traits that are causing symptoms related to Autonomic Overload Syndrome, rest assured that the success rate for your Combo personality in the Pain-Free for Life Program is the same as that of those who have only one personality type.

Finally, you should note that I referred to Erin's and my personality in the present tense. After you go through the Pain-Free for Life Program, you'll still have your same personality. The difference is that you'll learn how your personality causes dangerous emotions, and you'll learn to neutralize the harmful effects of repressed emotions on your body. You'll also begin to understand better how to identify the dangerous emotions as they're happening—to prevent a mountain of them from building up and overwhelming your autonomic nervous system again.

You should now be beginning to understand how your past experiences, present circumstances, and pain-prone personality all contribute to the mountain of strong repressed dangerous emotions that cause AOS. Next, I want to introduce you to another piece of the puzzle—the role of spirituality and spiritual health in the development of Autonomic Overload Syndrome.

But don't worry if you're not spiritually inclined. If you decide to steer clear of spirituality, you can be cured completely with the other mind–body treatments described in this book. But if you *do* have a spiritual bent, it will open the door to an even wider array of treatments—as well as a powerful means for you to *stay pain-free* after you complete the 6-week program.

THE SPIRITUAL
HEALTH INVENTORY
FOR PAIN

No one really knows the full extent to which spirituality impacts our health—and our pain. But there do seem to be significant connections among the mind, body, and spirit, as evidenced in studies consistently indicating that spiritual health has a positive effect on the health of the mind and body.

In my practice with AOS patients, more than two-thirds have expressed an interest in spirituality. Also, many have indicated that addressing their spiritual health has been an important part of their journey out of pain and into maintenance of a pain-free life.

Part of my preliminary examination of patients who have AOS pain involves taking an extensive spiritual history. In fact, it's been my experience that the level of spiritual health is an important factor in the development and treatment of AOS symptoms, and also can be a powerful aid in continuing to live pain-free. As far as AOS pain is concerned, spiritual health can be a factor on a par with the pain-prone personality, because spirituality often helps influence the level of dangerous negative emotions that are produced day in and day out.

But if you're not spiritually interested at all, please don't be put off as you begin this chapter, or feel in any way that this book is not for you. About one-third of my AOS patients are also not interested in spirituality or personal spiritual health; yet their recovery rates are high, similar to those who are spiritually inclined.

The spiritual component in AOS can emerge in a number of ways. For example, after recovery from AOS pain, many patients (including those not interested in spirituality) have called me and said something like this: "Dr. Brady, I'm amazed at the amounts of anger I've found in my subconscious mind—I had no idea! I'm also amazed at the levels of anger and other dangerous emotions that I feel every day. Will it always be like that? Is there something I can do to quit producing all these negative emotions?"

More often than not, I'll respond: "You're asking me a question that has spiritual implications. You see, spirituality is like a filter or buffer for the circumstances of the day. When you're spiritually healthy, you'll react differently to the circumstances and may produce lesser amounts of anger and other dangerous emotions. When you're spiritually unhealthy, or when you're not inclined toward spirituality at all, there's no buffer. In that case, you'll usually continue to produce and experience the same huge levels of dangerous emotions. But remember, whatever level of spirituality you have, just recognize—and don't repress—the dangerous emotions, and you'll be okay."

One reason I'm so adamant about injecting spirituality into the equation is the fact that scientific research is showing increasingly that the realm of the spirit can exert a tremendous influence on our health and well-being.

SPIRITUALITY AND HEALTH

Spirituality is an important part of most patients' lives. Polls consistently report that more than 90 percent of Americans believe in

God, and medical studies show that over 77 percent of patients want their physician to consider their spiritual needs during the medical encounter. In addition, spirituality and the interaction of mind, body, and spirit are increasingly being studied and reported in medical literature.

A Duke University study, for instance, showed that those who attended religious services at least once a week, and who prayed or studied the Bible at least daily, had consistently lower blood pressure than those who did so less frequently or not at all.[1]

Another Duke study demonstrated a 25 to 30 percent reduction in heart procedure complication rates when prayer and related responses were employed to reduce stress and anxiety. Furthermore, the lowest medical complication rates were observed in those patients assigned to off-site prayer sessions.[2]

In a similar vein, researchers from the Franklin Cardiac Rehabilitation Program in Franklin, North Carolina, studied participants of the Ornish Lifestyle Heart Trial to see if spirituality scores from a Spiritual Orientation Inventory correlated with progression or regression of coronary heart disease. These researchers found that the spirituality score correlated significantly with the degree of atherosclerotic coronary artery obstruction over a four-year period. Specifically, the lowest spiritual health scores had the *most progression* of coronary artery blockage, while the highest scores had the *most regression* of blockage. In other words, the study suggests that spiritual health may be an important factor in retarding and even reversing the development of coronary artery disease.

In confirmation of these scientific findings, Duke University physician and researcher Harold Koenig, editor of the *Handbook of Religion and Health*,[3] says that more than twelve hundred studies have now examined the relationship between religious involvement and various aspects of health. At least two-thirds of the studies evaluated have shown significant associations between religious activity and better mental and physical health. Some of these studies have indicated that spiritual and emotional health may help with:

- High blood pressure.
- Recovery after a heart attack.
- Immune system function.
- Depression.
- Chronic pain.
- Some types of arthritis.
- Your overall chances of dying.

In addition to the impact of spiritual health on physical disease, recent studies have also focused on the impact of spiritual health on pain.

THE SPIRIT–PAIN CONNECTION

A 2005 study[4] sponsored by Stanford University, ABC News, and *USA Today*, which dealt with the pain dilemma we face in America, has come up with some unexpected spiritual findings. According to this study, "*More than half of all Americans* are limping through life these days with the aggravation of on-again, off-again pain or the utter misery of hard-to-treat chronic pain. The result is less work, crankier mood and fewer activities, combined with a wide-ranging search for pain relief" (emphasis added).

The survey also made these findings:

- Back pain is by far the most common complaint, though knees and shoulders are also problems. About one-quarter of all the respondents cite back pain as their most recent difficulty, and another quarter cite joint pain.
- Attempted treatments include everything from over-the-counter drugs to alcohol. *But prayer and prescription drugs come out on top as most effective.*

In a classic description of chronic pain, the Stanford representatives said that people are "clear on where they hurt, but often can't link that pain to a specific cause." They also noted that *"in a surprising look at what works for pain relief, researchers find that just as many people cite prayers as prescription drugs"* (emphasis added).

It has been my experience that many (if not most) of these people studied by the Stanford researchers may be experiencing AOS pain and related symptoms. As a result, they would benefit from our 6-week Pain-Free for Life Program.

Finally, after surveying the medical literature that explores links between pain and spirituality, Dr. Harold Koenig and Duke University colleagues stated, "The evidence suggests an inverse relationship between pain intensity and both religious beliefs and religious attendance."[5] They noted that the findings were consistent with other research that has established a positive association between good physical health and religious faith and practice. But the discovery of the relationship of spiritual health to physical and emotional health is not new; it's been understood for many years.

ROOTS OF SPIRITUAL HEALING

For thousands of years, people in every culture have believed that physical health was influenced by emotional and spiritual health. For example, Solomon, another ancient Israelite king, highlighted this theme almost three thousand years ago in various passages in the proverbs.

In Proverbs 14:30 (HCSB), King Solomon advises that a "peaceful heart gives life to the body" while spiritually suspect emotions such as "jealousy" result in "rottenness to the bones." Later, he says, "A cheerful heart is good medicine, but a crushed spirit dries up the bones [or the body]" (17:22). In AOS terms, a crushed spirit might involve disappointment, anger, or grief.

Other proverbs of Solomon also warn specifically about the dangerous emotion of anger (29:11; 22:24–5; 19:19) and assert that those who are "slow to anger" are wise. Similarly, Solomon talks about the medical effects of shame, which—like jealousy—will also produce "rottenness" in the "bones" (12:4).

Like the Proverbs, the Psalms provide an especially useful model for linking dangerous emotions to spiritual and physical health. Consider again the words that Solomon's father, King David, wrote in Psalm 38 (NIV): "My guilt has overwhelmed me . . . My wounds fester . . . My back is filled with searing pain; there is no health in my body. . . . My strength fails me; even the light has gone from my eyes. . . . My pain is ever with me. . . . I confess my iniquity; I am troubled by my sin."

To put his observations in our terms, David was spiritually unhealthy; he felt distant from God, he felt extreme guilt, and he was experiencing searing back pain. What treatment did he choose? He certainly didn't resort to some tenth-century BC version of codeine or back surgery. Instead, he turned to a strong spiritual salve: confession of his guilt, coupled with prayer and a return to trust and faith in God. "Come quickly to help me, O Lord my Savior," he wrote.

Several factors seem to have been at work in producing relief from pain for these ancient writers, some of which we will introduce later on in the Pain-Free for Life Program. They understood the link between their symptoms and nonstructural causes (the mind–body–spirit link); they were able to identify the strong negative emotions by writing them out (depth journaling) and talking them out (pain talk); and finally, they renewed their connection with and trust in God (spiritual health).

This tradition continues into the early Christian experience recorded in the New Testament. For example, James gives some highly practical "how-to" spiritual healing advice in his epistle:

Is anyone among you suffering? He should pray. . . . Is anyone among you sick? He should call for the elders of the church, and they should pray over him after anointing him with olive oil in the name of the Lord. The prayer of faith will save the sick person, and the Lord will raise him up; and if he has committed sins, he will be forgiven. Therefore, confess your sins to one another and pray for one another so that you may be healed. (James 5:13–6, HCSB)

Here we have a treasure trove of mind–body–spirit healing guidelines. James advises *combining* individual prayer, group prayer, the presence of the divine (anointing with oil), and confession of guilt and wrongdoing. Another way of describing this healing experience is that if you're sick and experiencing pain, bring God into the equation through every mode of prayer available to you. Belief *plus* prayer *plus* confession *plus* fellowship with other believers make up an extremely strong healing potion.

After you begin the Pain-Free for Life Program, you may very well find that some of these old traditions like prayer, confession, and faith become increasingly important to you. This was certainly the experience of one of my patients, Annie.

ANNIE DISCOVERS A SPIRIT–PAIN LINK

Years before she came in to see me, Annie had gone in for an MRI because of a bout with severe lower back pain. In fact, she had undergone back surgery to get rid of that earlier pain, but she said, "My back never felt completely great."

Then Annie suffered another back injury when she was helping move a piano into her new home shortly after she had gotten married.

"I heard a pop, and maybe a month later, my back started to hurt," she said. "At the time, I attributed the pain to the piano incident."

The lower back pain flowed down her sciatic nerve into her left leg. She also suffered numbness and a tingling sensation, but mostly it was "just awful pain." An ardent athlete, she found that her regular jogging routine made her back pain worse; she even started to hurt when she sat still for a long time. Then the back pain extended into the times when she got up after she had been sitting. Finally, she began to hurt at night.

Gradually, Annie reduced her entire activity level, but the pain still grew worse. Another MRI revealed that she had two herniated disks, a condition that was consistent with the previous MRI taken almost ten years earlier.

Adamant about not having more surgery, and exhausted by the failure of traditional medicine to find an answer, Annie began to look toward mind–body solutions, including a program that had some similarities to my Pain-Free for Life Program. But even though she followed this program closely, her pain ultimately "got worse and worse. The pain was making me exceedingly depressed and frustrated. I was frustrated because I could not seem to conquer the pain and uncover the true source of my pain. I knew in my heart that the answer lay somewhere in the mind–body area, but I just couldn't make the pain go away."

Then she came in to see me. Here is her account of our appointment:

We sat down in his office and Dr. Brady began asking me about my life, questions no doctor had bothered to ask ever before. We talked about my marriage and how my efforts to keep the honeymoon going—by ignoring any frustrations and concerns—were causing a buildup of repressed emotions.

We talked about my self-sacrificing [People-Pleasing] and Perfectionist personality. Then we talked about God.

He asked me how I thought God viewed me and vice versa. I didn't think God thought too much of me. I saw God as a terrifying father figure, frowning down on me and making me take two steps backward from heaven for every bad thing I did in my life. This conversation was eye-opening for me, as I had not considered my spirituality—or my happy marriage—to be potential sources of my repressed emotions and pain.

Dr. Brady gave me a physical examination, reviewed my X-rays, and confirmed that none of my pain symptoms were attributed to a herniated disk. He also gave me a seminar [about chronic AOS pain] and shared medical evidence for his program and his own personal struggle and recovery from [chronic pain].

I left his office feeling freed of any lingering doubt about my diagnosis. And I became quite thoughtful about my spiritual background—how I was raised and how my People-Pleasing personality stemmed from my feelings of not being unconditionally loved and accepted by God. I was desperately seeking acceptance and approval from other people instead of God. I had been buried under a heavy blanket of guilt over not ever being good enough to others and not doing enough good things to please God.

When Annie returned home, she experienced instant success applying the Pain-Free Program techniques:

I had now fully accepted the diagnosis as real and had no remaining doubts. This was a key to my quick recovery. I read through Dr. Brady's seminar notes . . . and really just battled my brain for a while, especially when I would bend over or start running. As I began to hurt, I would just stop and say No! to myself. Then I'd bend over again. Almost always, the second time I had no pain. Or sometimes, I just ran through the pain and talked to myself, saying, "Stop hurting! There is no reason to have pain now!" And it would go away.

Within two weeks, Annie found she was free from pain, running regularly, doing yoga stretches, and engaging in activities she had been avoiding for almost two years. Since conquering the back pain, several other minor ailments and pains have cropped up. But:

I instantly know how to cure them. I think about what might be bothering me and how it threatens my self-image. I also write about my repressed emotions in a journal when I feel symptoms coming on. Then I promptly turn my thoughts to something else and pay no mind to the ailment. It always goes away in a matter of minutes, or a couple of days.

Annie has taken no medicine in years, not even an aspirin. Furthermore, health problems that had plagued her before—such as yeast infections, sinus infections, headaches, and backaches—have disappeared.

Perhaps her most telling insight involves a profound spiritual understanding about herself and her pain:

My journey through pain and recovery was really God using pain in my life to show me that my life was off track. I was not living the life that He intended for me. I truly believe that God uses pain and suffering to bring us closer to Him. I see it (my pain) as an incredible blessing that has made me a better person in every way. He wanted to take me higher and release me from the guilt I had labored under for so many years. My pain came at a time when I didn't know who I was if I couldn't do something to get approval from others. It came at a time when I was needing to turn the page from being a girl controlled by everyone else's expectations to becoming a woman who knows what she wants and needs to be happy.

The discussions with Dr. Brady about my views of God led me to deeply examine my religious background. I began reading the Bible in order to separate the truth from what others had taught me to believe. Now I have a close, more personal and unconditionally loving relationship with God. As a result, our happy marriage is just that: much happier and more honest and fulfill-ing. My life in general is much more honest and fulfilling.

It's impossible to add anything of significance to such accounts of recovery, except to note that—for Annie, myself, and so many others who have recovered from AOS pain—the Pain-Free for Life Program has been a path to wholeness: a healing of mind and body and spirit.

Now let's get a little more specific about exactly what "spiritual health" is and how it may affect your AOS symptoms.

SPIRITUALITY AND SPIRITUAL HEALTH

Spirituality involves a transcendent experience, which often brings into play the emotions, thoughts, and behavior. This topic is often difficult to discuss because of the personal and indefinable nature of faith and experience. To facilitate understanding and free discussion, it can be helpful from the outset to differentiate between spirituality and ordinary religion (or "religiousness")—factors that have a direct bearing on your spiritual health or spiritual distress, and your pain.

More specifically, when I talk with patients about the meaning of true spirituality and good spiritual health, I like to distinguish between *intrinsic spirituality* and *extrinsic spirituality* or religiousness.[6] Those who are intrinsically spiritual are typically deeply influenced in their daily decision making, attitudes, and actions by their spiritual convictions. For example, this kind of person might be inclined to read Scripture and meditate throughout the week, pray about small and large decisions, and understand the meaning of life in terms of his or her relationship to God.

In contrast, those who are extrinsically spiritual or religious tend to feature the outward behaviors of belief—such as membership in a religious organization or strict adherence to attendance or ritual.

But their involvement remains a surface affair rather than a personal experience or an affair of the heart. With extrinsic spirituality, or religiousness, personal beliefs tend not to influence daily actions, decisions, or a worldview to any degree.

While intrinsic spirituality is by nature deeply personal and experiential, religiousness or extrinsic spirituality may focus on a specific set of beliefs, teachings, and practices without leading to intrinsic spirituality. In many of my AOS patients, this kind of religion has led to much spiritual distress (or spiritual unhealthiness), with teachings that lead more often to stressful pressure than to freedom . . . to guilt rather than to forgiveness . . . and to pretending rather than honesty.

As I've indicated, about two-thirds of my AOS patients describe themselves as spiritual, saying that their interest in spiritual things ranks at least a seven on a scale of one through ten, with ten being the highest level of spiritual interest. I've found that, within that same group, when I ask them questions about their level of spiritual health (as reflected in the Spiritual Inventory later in this chapter), relatively few end up considering themselves "spiritually healthy." My conclusion from a health perspective is this: Being spiritual is better than being religious. But being spiritual doesn't guarantee that you're spiritually healthy; it just means that your faith is very important and deeply personal to you.

In a 2001 *American Family Practice* article, Brown University physicians Hight and Anandarajah describe spiritual health as "the experiential and emotional aspects involving feelings of hope, love, connection, inner peace, comfort and support. These are reflected in the quality of the individual's inner resources, the ability to give and receive spiritual love, and the types of relationships and connections that exist with self, community . . . and the transcendent."[7]

In my practice, I've defined spiritual health this way:

Spiritual health *refers to a connectedness and trust in God
that involves confession, forgiveness, and belief—and results in
hope, peace, comfort, meaning, and a release from guilt, fear,
and pressure.*

According to the same *American Family Physician* article cited earlier, the opposite of spiritual health is spiritual distress—a condition in which individuals are generally unable consistently to find sources of meaning, hope, love, peace, comfort, strength, or connection in life. Also, spiritual distress may arise when significant conflict occurs between our deepest beliefs and what is actually happening in our lives. Such distress can have a detrimental effect on physical and mental health.[8]

To put these distinctions still another way, you may consider yourself spiritual rather than religious, but you probably won't be considered spiritually healthy unless your faith gives you a pervasive and predominant sense of

- Hope instead of fear.
- Love instead of condemnation.
- Inner peace instead of anxiety.
- Comfort instead of inner turmoil.
- Connection with God instead of isolation and loneliness.
- Meaning in life instead of meaninglessness.
- Assurance about your life instead of doubt and uncertainty.

These subjective qualities are part of the inner transcendent experience that makes up true spiritual health. Also, in my experience, spiritual health is a lot like physical health: It comes and goes, is never perfect, and can always improve. And when we are most spiritually healthy, we're more likely to experience emotional, psychological, and physical health as well.

But how specifically does all this relate to pain—and especially *your* pain? To begin to answer this question, let me walk you through a typical scenario.

A Spiritual Health Scenario

Generally speaking, intrinsic spirituality serves as a powerful filter or buffer that sifts the circumstances and stresses of each day. The same stressful circumstances will result in lower production of strong negative emotions if the spiritual health buffer or filter is stronger.

As shown below (figure E), our spiritual health diverts or neutralizes the impact of stressful daily circumstances.

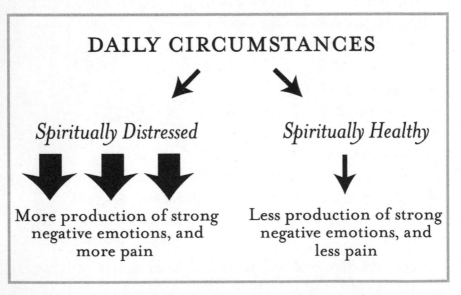

Figure E

Here's how the sequence of events shown in this graph may work in practice. I've chosen examples of two AOS patients responding to the same stressful circumstance:

Stressful Circumstance:

❖ The stock market and your retirement investments take a large tumble as the market crashes five thousand points in one day.

Spirituality Filter:

Person 1 (in spiritual distress) believes: "I am in control—the pressure is on *me*. If anything in life is going to go right, it's because *I* work for it and *I* deserve it. I'm ultimately responsible for the outcome of my life."

(His spirituality—or lack thereof—is defined by fear, pressure, anxiety, and isolation.)

Person 2 (excellent spiritual health) believes: "I'm not alone. God is in control of every circumstance of my life. Things don't always work out the way I want. But I believe He works everything out for my good because He really loves me. He's *for* me."

(Her intrinsic spirituality is defined by hope, inner peace, comfort, and connection with God.)

Emotional Response:
Response of Person 1:
❖ Anger, shock, fear, and anxiety at the situation.
❖ Building anger—and rage—at being out of control and under so much pressure.
❖ Waves of anxiety and fear because of the uncertainty of his future.
❖ Fear and pressure because his situation is completely up to him.
❖ Guilt and shame because he should have been smarter with the money.

Response of Person 2:

- Initial disappointment, anxiety, fear, and anger—similar to Person 1, but maybe a bit less intense.
- A growing sense of comfort and strength and security through her trust in God: "It's scary, but I know God will take care of me. God is *for* me."
- A steadily increasing peace through prayer as her faith in God results in hope and comfort.
- Diminishing anxiety and anger as her connection with God brings transcendent strength, peace, and assurance of the future.

Wrapping Up the Scenario

Although the circumstances were the same, Person 1 experienced the physical symptoms of back tightness and a headache. But Person 2 displayed no physical symptoms. Why? Because the same circumstances were filtered through different spiritual health filters, the emotional responses were different. Consequently, the physical effects due to the level of repressed emotions were also different.

Now let's take a closer look at a process I use at the Brady Institute to help determine the level of spiritual health of my AOS patients.

IT'S TIME FOR *YOUR* SPIRITUAL HEALTH INVENTORY

As I've mentioned, I take a spiritual history on all patients I'm examining for AOS pain and related symptoms. Although there are many different types of spiritual health inventories, I've created my own inventory around the HOPE format offered to physicians by Drs. Anandarajah and Hight in their 2001 *American Family Physician* article. *HOPE* is an acronym for a four-category approach to asking patients about spirituality:

H: Ask about sources of **H**ope, strength, comfort, meaning, peace, love, and connection.

O: Ask about the role of **O**rganized religion for the patient.

P: Ask about **P**ersonal spirituality and practices.

E: Ask about the **E**ffects of a patient's spirituality and beliefs on medical care and end-of-life issues.

With this in mind, pretend you're in my office and we're progressing through your history. We've covered your current pain complaints, your past medical history, your previous surgeries and medications, and your family and social history. We've just finished talking about your pain-prone personality style, your fears of any activities, and any stressful events you can remember from your past and present circumstances. Now it's time for me to take your spiritual history.

To get an idea about the current state of your spiritual health, and how that health may be affecting your pain, I want you to take the Spiritual Health Inventory for Pain reproduced on pages 142 to 145. The list of questions will give you a sense if you're spiritually healthy or in spiritual distress. Those who are in spiritual distress sometimes discover that their spiritual unhealthiness is actually contributing significantly to the onslaught of dangerous repressed emotions, which results in AOS pain.

As you jot down your answers to the following questions, you may want to use a separate journal for your responses—both to give yourself plenty of space to answer and also to get started with the depth-journaling strategy that we'll discuss in detail in chapter 9. Feel free to skip questions that you feel don't apply to you.

If you feel a particular question doesn't apply to you, leave it blank. Above all, be honest. No one needs to see these responses except you.

THE SPIRITUAL HEALTH INVENTORY FOR PAIN

Part 1: Sources of Hope, Meaning, Comfort, Strength, Peace, Love, and Connection

	NO/ NEVER	RARELY	SOMETIMES	USUALLY	YES/ ALWAYS
1. Do you believe in God, or a Supreme Power?	1	2	3	4	5
2. Do you feel you have a personal relationship with God?	1	2	3	4	5

(3–10) Does your faith or trust in God give you:	NO/ NEVER	RARELY	SOMETIMES	USUALLY	YES/ ALWAYS
3. A pervasive sense of HOPE?	1	2	3	4	5
4. A pervasive sense of LOVE?	1	2	3	4	5
5. A pervasive sense of INNER PEACE?	1	2	3	4	5
6. A pervasive sense of COMFORT?	1	2	3	4	5
7. A pervasive sense of MEANING?	1	2	3	4	5
8. A pervasive sense of STRENGTH outside your own power?	1	2	3	4	5
9. A pervasive sense of CONNECTION WITH GOD?	1	2	3	4	5
10. A pervasive sense of CONFIDENCE in the future?	1	2	3	4	5

	NO/ NEVER	RARELY	SOMETIMES	USUALLY	YES/ ALWAYS
11. During your chronic pain, do you turn to God for comfort?	1	2	3	4	5
12. During stressful and hard times, do you feel God's peace?	1	2	3	4	5
13. Does prayer result in you feeling relaxed and at peace?	1	2	3	4	5
14. Do you feel loved and unconditionally accepted by God?	1	2	3	4	5
15. Do you often feel close to God?	1	2	3	4	5

Part 2: Organized Religion

	NO/ NEVER	RARELY	SOMETIMES	USUALLY	YES/ ALWAYS
16. Are you a member of a particular church, synagogue, mosque, or other religious group?	1	2	3	4	5
17. Do you attend religious services weekly?	1	2	3	4	5

(18–20) Does your religion generally cause you to be:	NO/ NEVER	RARELY	SOMETIMES	USUALLY	YES/ ALWAYS
18. Less judgmental (critical) than most people?	1	2	3	4	5
19. Less irritated with others of different beliefs?	1	2	3	4	5
20. More loving toward people in general?	1	2	3	4	5

	NO/ NEVER	RARELY	SOMETIMES	USUALLY	YES/ ALWAYS
21. Do you have close relationships with people within your particular place of worship?	1	2	3	4	5
22. Do you participate in any organized fellowship groups with those in your religious community?	1	2	3	4	5
23. When you're around people from your religious community are you generally honest and open discussing your feelings and personal issues (versus quiet or pretending all is okay)?	1	2	3	4	5

(24–30) Do the teachings of your organized religion tend to:	NO/ NEVER	RARELY	SOMETIMES	USUALLY	YES/ ALWAYS
24. Make you feel UNBURDENED (versus obligated and heavy)?	1	2	3	4	5
25. Make you feel FORGIVEN (versus guilty)?	1	2	3	4	5
26. Make you feel FREE (versus under pressure)?	1	2	3	4	5
27. Make you feel ENCOURAGED (versus discouraged)?	1	2	3	4	5
28. Make you feel LOVED by God (versus judged)?	1	2	3	4	5

	NO/ NEVER	RARELY	SOMETIMES	USUALLY	YES/ ALWAYS
29. Make you feel HOPEFUL about the future (versus fearful)?	1	2	3	4	5
30. Make you feel CONCERNED with others (versus angry)?	1	2	3	4	5

Part 3: Personal Spirituality and Practices

	NO/ NEVER	RARELY	SOMETIMES	USUALLY	YES/ ALWAYS
31. Do you have an active faith in God?	1	2	3	4	5
32. Is your faith PERSONAL (versus abstract, impersonal)?	1	2	3	4	5
33. Is your faith GROWING (versus stagnant or diminishing)?	1	2	3	4	5
34. Is your faith VITAL to you (versus going through the motions)?	1	2	3	4	5
35. Is your faith in God IMPORTANT to you?	1	2	3	4	5

(36–40) What is your view of God?	NO/ NEVER	RARELY	SOMETIMES	USUALLY	YES/ ALWAYS
36. God is patient and difficult to anger	1	2	3	4	5
37. God is kind and generous to me personally	1	2	3	4	5
38. God is concerned about me individually	1	2	3	4	5
39. God is loving and He loves me unconditionally	1	2	3	4	5
40. God is forgiving and He forgives me quickly	1	2	3	4	5

	NO/ NEVER	RARELY	SOMETIMES	USUALLY	YES/ ALWAYS
41. Is your faith more important to you NOW than in the past?	1	2	3	4	5
42. Do you engage in personal confession frequently?	1	2	3	4	5
43. Do you engage in private prayer frequently?	1	2	3	4	5
44. Do you ever pray corporately or in groups?	1	2	3	4	5
45. Do you usually pray about OTHERS' needs (versus your own)?	1	2	3	4	5

	NO/ NEVER	RARELY	SOMETIMES	USUALLY	YES/ ALWAYS
46. When you pray, do you believe God is actually listening?	1	2	3	4	5
47. Do you engage in private meditation or reflection about God?	1	2	3	4	5
48. Do you think more about what God thinks of you (versus what others think about you)?	1	2	3	4	5
49. In general, do you rely heavily on God to live out each day?	1	2	3	4	5
50. Do you find that you are quick to forgive others?	1	2	3	4	5

Part 4: Effects of Spirituality on Your Medical Condition

	NO/ NEVER	RARELY	SOMETIMES	USUALLY	YES/ ALWAYS
51. Has your struggle with chronic pain generally ENHANCED your spirituality and personal beliefs?	1	2	3	4	5
52. When you have pain, do you often ask others to pray for you?	1	2	3	4	5
53. Despite your pain, have you been able to take steps or do things that help you spiritually?	1	2	3	4	5
54. Are you now looking (or thinking about looking) for ways that might help you reconnect with your spiritual community?	1	2	3	4	5
55. Are you now looking (or thinking about looking) for ways that might help you reconnect with God?	1	2	3	4	5

TOTAL SCORE_____ (275 possible)

<100: You may be in SIGNIFICANT Spiritual DISTRESS.
100–165: You may be in MODERATE Spiritual DISTRESS.
166–230: You may have MODERATE Spiritual HEALTH.
>230: You may be enjoying SIGNIFICANT Spiritual HEALTH.

SUGGESTED ANSWER KEY

Although it's impossible in such a short space to do a definitive spiritual evaluation of anyone, the following guidelines may help you understand the current state of your spiritual health—and what you might do to improve that health. Also, as you total up your answers and match them against the scale below, remember that the purpose of this little exercise is to give you a better idea of your spiritual strengths—and how they might be employed to deal with your AOS pain.

First, add up all your scores on the questions you answered. If you left a question blank, count that response as a 0. You'll see that the highest score you could achieve on the inventory is 275, but I certainly don't expect anyone to hit that mark. As indicated below, any score above 165 qualifies as moderate spiritual health.

In any case, here are some *suggested* ranges about what those scores may mean.

- **Less than 100.** You may be in severe spiritual distress. In other words, you have virtually no spiritual buffer standing between your daily stresses and the strong daily negative emotions that result.
- **100–165.** You may be in moderate spiritual distress.
- **166–230.** You may be in moderate spiritual health.
- **>230.** You may be enjoying significant spiritual health. In other words, you appear to have strong spiritual buffers for life's circumstances and stresses. Also, you may tend to produce fewer and less intense negative emotions than most people as a result of life events. Finally, your spiritual buffer can be a great asset as you try to maintain a pain-free life. But remember that spiritual health by itself isn't enough. You must learn how to *employ your spiritual strengths* in combating your pain.

The answers to the above inventory questions should give you a good start in determining your current level of spiritual health. As you continue your spiritual journey—exploring how your insights may be applied in dealing with dangerous emotions and AOS pain—keep in mind that there is really no single spiritual technique or strategy that will apply to everyone. But I believe that it is important for each of us to recognize that we are made up of mind, body, and spirit. In other words, we are spiritual beings, meant to be connected to God and experience spiritual health.

In the end, my best advice would be to ask you to keep in mind the definition of spiritual health that I gave you earlier:

Spiritual health refers to a connectedness and trust in God
that involves confession, forgiveness, and belief—and results
in hope, peace, comfort, meaning, and a release from guilt, fear,
and pressure.

With this understanding always in sharp focus—and with a commitment to make the different parts of the definition a reality in your life—you'll be more likely to stay on the path that leads to spiritual health.

Furthermore, as your spiritual health improves, you'll find that you have fewer strong negative emotions to deal with—or repress—because you perceive your circumstances and stresses differently. Instead of feeling alone, scared, or angry, you will start to discover that your trust in God is allowing you to rest and experience transcendent peace and comfort at a different level. Such inner changes will give you an advantage in maintaining the pain-free life. Of course, no one will become a perfect spiritual being in this life. But spiritual perfection is not the goal; maximum spiritual health is. So, wherever you are in your spiritual life, be assured that you can develop further—and resolve to take the next step.

THE ROOTS OF
MIND–BODY–SPIRIT
MEDICINE

By now, you may be wondering how the medical field got to this point . . . a point where holistic approaches to disease and pain are uncommon . . . a point where physicians usually look at their patients through the very narrow lens of body medicine . . . and a point where most of my patients ask, "Hey, how come my doctor never mentioned this mind–body stuff?"

How exactly *did* medicine get here—and what can we expect in the future?

For thousands of years, the physician–patient encounter involved the whole person: body, mind, and spirit. Physical ailments were investigated with a holistic approach. Patients were understood to be spiritual, psychological, and physical beings—and the best medical treatments involved an analysis of all three. In the words of one of the history's most respected physicians, Sir William Osler, "While the good physician treats the disease, the great physician treats the patient"—meaning the *whole* patient.

It's only been in the past 150 years or so that holistic evaluation and treatment has been nudged out by the narrow mechanistic view of illness. Now, it's my opinion that the era of modern, mechanistic body medicine has been a wonderful and necessary step in the advancement of healing. The mechanistic/body era has advanced our understanding of the physical body by leaps and bounds. We've gone from superstition to fact, and from guessing to evidence. Yet we've lost the whole person in the process.

But now we're returning to a more holistic understanding in medicine. Ever so slowly, holistic medicine is finding its way back in published research, medical school training, clinical practice, and even government funding through the National Institutes of Health. Although your doctor might not be there yet, holistic evaluation and treatment paradigms are ushering in a new medicine— an approach in which the good things about the old medicine are added to what is true about modern medicine. When these forces come together, the possibilities for discovery and cure are staggering. So let's take a look back at the exciting history of mind–body–spirit medicine: where we've come, where we are, and where we may be going in designing the most effective treatments for your pain.

Body Medicine: New Kid on the Block

Evidence that mind–body–spirit strategies actually work in treating Autonomic Overload Syndrome pain can be found in the long, exciting history of mind–body medicine. In fact, the mind–body–spirit links to your AOS pain have been accumulating and strengthening for many years. It's only recently that mechanistic/body medicine has taken over the medical world (at least in Western society), ushering in tremendous advances in our understanding of sickness and health, including:

- The eradication of smallpox through the work of Edward Jenner in the 1800s.

- Antiseptic surgery introduced in the mid-1800s by Louis Pasteur, who said that airborne microbes could cause disease (by the way, he was vilified by the medical establishment at the time).
- Robert Koch's identification of tuberculosis and anthrax.
- The discovery of antiseptics and techniques for cleanliness through the work of Joseph Lister.
- The accidental discovery of the X-ray by Wilhelm Roentgen in 1893, which later led to the development of the CT scanner and the MRI.
- The development of aspirin in 1897 by Bayer and the chemist Hoffman in a personal quest to relieve a father's arthritic pain.
- The discovery of penicillin by Alexander Fleming in 1928.
- The development of vaccines and a wide array of antibiotics that can prevent and cure once deadly infections such as polio, tetanus, and pneumonia.
- The development of thousands of pharmaceutical medicines to help life-threatening conditions, including diabetes, hypertension, and congestive heart failure.
- Cancer treatments including chemotherapy and radiation therapy.
- Advanced surgery, which can replace vessels of the heart, transplant major organs, and replace worn-out joints including hips and knees.

The mechanistic/body era of medicine has seen 150 years of magnificence; but in light of the history of medicine, it's clearly the new kid on the block.

MEDICINE'S BIRTH IN THE MIND AND SPIRIT

For most of human history, mind–body–spirit treatments occupied the premier position in the average healer's toolbox. In part this approach emerged because physicians didn't have many alternatives; but for the most part, early physicians turned to mind–body–spirit treatments because their philosophy of medicine was holistic. Until recently, medicine has always treated the patient as a whole, and tried to understand the nature of illness from a holistic perspective.

Most ancient healing practices, such as traditional Chinese medicine and ayurvedic medicine, have always emphasized the important links between mind and body. In fact, the ancient art of acupuncture, which has recently made its way onto the stage of Western medicine, takes into account mind–body interactions to increase blood flow to painful parts (sound familiar?).

Similarly, meditative techniques have been used for millennia in various cultures to calm the mind and spirit, ward off pain, reduce stress, and control various bodily functions. The psalmist Aspah complained of depression, weakness of spirit, and insomnia in Psalm 77. Then he found the treatment: "At night I remember my music; I meditate in my heart, and my spirit ponders" (Psalm 77:6, HCSB).

But in some ways, talking about ancient medicine begs the question: Are there really any measurable health benefits that flow from such practices? In an effort to answer this and related questions, a team of researchers from Harvard Medical School used thermometers and other modern medical technology to test the physical responses of a group of Tibetan Buddhist monks who used meditative mind–body techniques that had been devised centuries earlier.

The researchers, led by Dr. Herbert Benson, found that by the application of their mind–body techniques, monks experienced reduced heart rates; lower blood pressure; and increased skin temperatures (up to fifteen degrees Fahrenheit), which enabled them to calm their minds and bodies and withstand painfully cold temperatures (forty degrees) while wrapped in cold, wet sheets. Those from other philosophical and religious traditions, including both

Catholicism and Protestantism, have used their own meditative practices to reduce high blood pressure, eliminate various physical pains, and achieve other health benefits.[1]

A basic principle underlying such ancient mind–body medical traditions—one recognized increasingly by contemporary, scientifically grounded mind–body research—is the God-given healing power of nature and the body. This concept, recognized in the fourth century BC,[2] by the ancient Greek founder of modern medicine, Hippocrates, is based on the assumption that the human body contains innate capacities to heal itself and achieve freedom from pain. The challenge for the physician was to help the patient identify these natural capacities and exploit and release them to produce a cure whenever possible, without resorting to invasive medical techniques.

One important way that patients through the centuries have accessed this natural healing power has been to learn ways to unmask strong negative emotions, which have long been linked to pain and disease. In this vein, Hippocrates is said to have told his patients suffering from asthma that they should beware of anger.[3] More recently, Fred Luskin and lead researcher Carl Thoreson at Stanford University addressed the harmful effects of negative emotions in the Forgiveness Study, which tested the ability of forgiveness to help ailments including hypertension, pain, and other stress-related disorders. The outcomes have been quite successful, and the practice of forgiveness has led to many physical and emotional health benefits by decreasing dangerous, stress-related emotions such as anger and anxiety.

Yet these strong beginnings in mind–body–spirit medicine were forgotten for a time with the rise of a body-medicine bias. This bias, which still exerts powerful influence in our own time, has to be confronted directly by anyone who hopes to experience maximum benefits from a mind–body–spirit approach to pain relief.

THE ASCENT OF SCIENCE

The pivotal misstep leading to the temporary end of holistic medicine took place in the seventeenth century with the famous French mathematician, scientist, and philosopher René Descartes. Descartes's entry onto the Western intellectual scene changed attitudes toward science and medicine decisively.

The father of Cartesian dualism or the mind–body split,[4] he proposed the idea that the mind and body should be separate and distinct because he couldn't understand how the soul (mind, spirit, and emotions) could interact with the body. The two to him seemed completely separate and different.

As a result of Descartes's insights, the body became an independent entity, which was placed under the purview of science and medicine. Later thinkers split off matters of the soul (including mind, spirit, and emotions) and put them exclusively in the care of religion and the clergy. This mind–body split ended holistic medical evaluation and treatment—including the evaluation and treatment of pain—for several hundred years.

Descartes himself explored the pain implications of his philosophy when, in 1664, he described what to this day is still called a pain pathway. In his exploration of this early medical theory, he illustrated how the sensations caused by particles of fire that came into contact with the foot could travel to the brain. In other words, his pain pathway was all about nerves running up to the brain and back down to the foot—classic body medicine.

By the nineteenth century, physical science began to take over pain therapy. Physician-scientists discovered that opium, morphine, codeine, and cocaine could be used to reduce or eliminate feelings of pain, at least for a limited time. About that same time, aspirin was discovered and became a medication that to this day is the most commonly used pain reliever.

Later, physicians refined the application of both general and regional anesthesia to eliminate pain as a major factor during surgery. Also, scientists discovered antibiotics, which, among other things, reduced the pain that occurred during infection. Before long, these giant strides in body medicine convinced most doctors and patients that the panacea for pain could be found in a prescription, an over-the-counter bottle, or a surgeon's scalpel.

As the scientific breakthroughs accelerated, medical practitioners rejected as old-fashioned the various mind–body–spirit strategies for healing pain. Medical schools taught anatomy and physiology with no consideration of mind, thoughts, emotions, or spiritual health on the physical condition. Consequently, physicians for years have blindly (and unknowingly) accepted, practiced, and taught each other a medical paradigm based on Descartes's notion of mind–body separation.

In practical terms, what this means is that for several generations, Western-trained physicians have not been able to understand how to explain chronic pain or other physical illnesses (including fibromyalgia, chronic back pain, irritable bowel syndrome, and various AOS symptoms) in any other terms except the standard body explanation.

Many patients, however, have not welcomed the results. By 1998, more than 40 percent of Americans had used complementary and alternative medicine, with an estimated six hundred million patient visits (most of which were concealed from their regular physician) and $27 billion in expenses. There was one main reason for this patient exodus from body medicine—it didn't work.[5]

Only recently have the proponents of body science begun to realize that the optimum treatment for many illnesses, including pain, may involve a more comprehensive and holistic approach—borrowing from what is old, and applying it to what is new.

THE REBIRTH OF MIND–BODY–SPIRIT MEDICINE

Ironically, the center of the rebirth of mind–body–spirit medicine—Boston and Cambridge, Massachusetts—is also a stronghold of important body-medicine research. The prestigious *New England Journal of Medicine* has its offices there. So does the Harvard Medical School, which thrives on sponsoring the latest medical research and turning out physicians who practice body medicine with the latest knowledge of drugs and surgery. But something else is going on at Harvard—a countertrend in treatment that reaches well back into the nineteenth century.

THE HARVARD TRADITION

The recent roots of the contemporary mind–body–spirit movement—and its use in treating pain—can be traced in part to a line of researchers at the Harvard Medical School, beginning in the mid–nineteenth century with the great professor of anatomy and physiology Oliver Wendell Holmes.[6]

Holmes, who also made his mark as an acclaimed writer and essayist, recognized and advocated scientific medical methodology, such as following sanitary practices in the hospital to prevent the spread of disease and infection. But at the same time, he acknowledged the ancient mind–body traditions of medicine. Among other things, he taught that a patient's personal beliefs and a caregiver's positive bedside manner could help the healing process.

In the latter part of the nineteenth century, the physician-psychologist-philosopher William James took Holmes's contributions a step farther: He began to conduct experiments that connected physiology, psychology, and spiritual experience. His research suggested that, when a particular idea became firmly fixed in a person's belief system, uncomfortable or even painful physical symptoms might result, such as choking, paralysis, bleeding, or tightening of muscles and tendons. Conversely, when the subjects were influenced to think positive, healing thoughts, the symptoms might disappear immediately. James discussed his idea of "Mind Cures" in his landmark book *The Varieties of Religious Experience.*

(As I reflect on these symptoms—and especially on the tightening of muscles and tendons—I'm reminded of many of my own patients who complain of various muscle pains, including chronic back pain and fibromyalgia. Yet they are cured with the mind–body–spirit interventions discussed later in the Pain-Free Program.)

One of William James's most attentive students was Walter Cannon, who graduated from medical school in 1900. He became the leading professor of physiology at Harvard in the first half of the twentieth century. Most important of all for our purposes, Cannon went on to identify the stress response to fear and danger, which is now known popularly as the fight-or-flight response.

Cannon's findings laid the groundwork for the now accepted insight that emotional pressures or traumas can produce excessive amounts of stress hormones and neurotransmitters, including epinephrine (adrenaline), norepinephrine, and cortisol. These biochemical responses can, in excess, lead to severe pain, cardiovascular disease, weight gain, fatigue, and a host of other health problems.

One of Cannon's medical students, A. Clifford Barger, carried on the tradition of linking body medicine to other disciplines. An expert on cardiovascular disorders, he believed that medicine should be approached as a whole-body enterprise—with the possibility that the operations of the mind might interact with body functions and health. This orientation intrigued one of Barger's students at the Harvard Medical School, Herbert Benson, who became a cardiologist and one of the pioneers of mind–body medicine.

In the late 1960s, Benson noticed in his research that the blood pressure of patients often rose when they were measured in a doctor's office; he suspected that the cause was related to increased stress. In other words, he had found an explanation for the phenomenon now known as "white coat hypertension"—when the doctor's office and sight of the physician's white coat heightens the patient's anxiety, along with blood pressure readings.

Finally, Benson's stress research enabled him to identify the relaxation response, the physiological opposite of the stress response.[7] The relaxation response—which has been associated with relief of pain in addition to many other health benefits—may be triggered by a variety of relaxation-enhancing techniques and exercises that we discuss in this book, including spiritual disciplines such as prayer. This process is typically accompanied by lower blood pressure, reduced heart rate, and slower breathing. As these biochemical and physiological changes related to parasympathetic activation occur, the patient begins to enjoy a greater sense of relaxation, less pain, less anxiety and depression, and relief from many negative emotions, including anger.

As these mind–body breakthroughs unfolded, several other important medical trends were moving forward in the 1970s and 1980s—sparked by Dr. Elmer Green's work with biofeedback, Dr. Candace B. Pert's research into the molecular foundations of our emotions, and Dr. John E. Sarno's therapeutic emphasis on unconscious emotions as a cause of chronic muscle pain.

BIOFEEDBACK

In 1970, Dr. Elmer Green and his wife introduced the concept of autogenic feedback—later known as biofeedback. Biofeedback is a mind–body technique in which people are trained to control their involuntary responses through their conscious thoughts. In other words, things normally under the control of our autonomic nervous system, such as blood pressure and heart rate, can be brought under voluntary control through mind–body training. Biofeedback has been used successfully for many conditions including tension headaches, migraine headaches, and chronic pain.

MOLECULES OF EMOTION

Dr. Candace Pert of the Georgetown University Medical Center (formerly with the NIH) is a leading researcher into human neuropeptides and receptors. By identifying what she calls the "molecules of emotion,"[8] Pert has made giant strides in the science of mind–body interactions that link the mind (thoughts, emotions) to the body.

In the early 1970s, Pert identified a receptor on the surface of cells that locks onto morphine-like molecules known as endorphins. These molecules have been associated with the so-called runner's high and other feelings of happiness. In nonmedical terms, she found a "baseball glove" (the specific receptor on the cell surface) where the endorphin molecule of happiness (the "baseball") fit perfectly. When this endorphin molecule—a molecule of emotion—is attached to the cell receptor in the brain, you experience bliss.

But Pert also found that endorphin receptors weren't just located in the brain; they are also found in the muscles, heart, intestines, and other organs. The implications are that your emotions don't affect just your brain, but your heart and intestines and muscles as well. Not only this, but Pert found receptors for other emotional molecules, including molecules of anger, fear, and sadness. In fact, almost every cell of our body is studded with thousands of receptors (baseball gloves) just waiting for a molecule of emotion to attach; and when it does, it changes the performance of the cell.

As Pert's research progressed, she concluded that stress impedes the free movement of various molecules of emotion in the human body. When these molecules of emotion are impeded, the unhealthy, repressed molecules stick around and are actually *stored* in the molecular receptors. But when an individual is able to pull long-buried negative emotions into consciousness through such strategies as controlled breathing, visualization, meditation, psychotherapy, or self-analysis, Pert says, the molecules of emotion begin flowing again—with a resulting improvement in emotional and physical health.

Despite Pert's fine work, along with that of other mind–body researchers, a major challenge remains: How can we apply the emerging research to relieve pain? The work of Dr. John E. Sarno of the Rusk Institute in Manhattan has moved us several steps closer to answering this question.

SARNO AND THE UNCONSCIOUS

Dr. John E. Sarno is physician and professor emeritus in the Department of Rehabilitation Medicine at NYU Medical Center. Over the past thirty years, he has designed a program that has been instrumental in helping many patients, including me, overcome chronic pain.

In the mid-1970s, Sarno noticed that many patients who experienced back pain, and who were being evaluated for possible back surgery, seemed to improve when they began to identify long-repressed stressful emotions. He coined the term *Tension Myositis Syndrome*, or TMS,[9] to refer to a group of painful conditions. In an explanation consistent with clinical research findings of Candace Pert and others, he believes that TMS begins with the repression (or burying in the unconscious mind) of destructive emotions, especially anger and unconscious rage.

I am indebted to Dr. Sarno for contributing to my physical cure and for "curing" my narrow Cartesian paradigm. In my practice with AOS, I've tried to build upon the wisdom of Drs. Sarno, Pert, and the "Harvard gang" while broadening my treatment strategies to include the lost spiritual dimension of the pain-free life. Over the years, I've developed a specific set of treatment steps that patients have successfully used to free themselves from chronic and debilitating AOS pain. These treatments are the core of my 6-week Pain-Free for Life Program, which is the subject of part 2 of this book.

PART TWO

THE PAIN-FREE FOR LIFE PROGRAM

THE 6-WEEK
PAIN-FREE FOR LIFE
TREATMENT PROGRAM

This program has been designed for use by all those who suffer chronic pain and symptoms related to the Autonomic Overload Syndrome. In this chapter, I'll introduce you in some detail to the 6-week Pain-Free for Life Program that I have developed—and used with considerable success—at the Brady Institute for Health. But first, here is a quick review of the pain conditions and symptoms that this program has been designed to remedy:

With AOS, painful physical symptoms occur as repressed emotions, stress, and pressure activate your autonomic nervous system. This system is turned on by your subconscious mind, and your repressed dangerous emotions keep it turned on. The subconscious mind also acts as the storehouse of these dangerous repressed emotions.

With chronic autonomic nervous system overactivation, you may experience various physical symptoms, including many types of chronic pain (see chapter 3)—*all* of which are treated with this 6-week program. These physical symptoms are, in effect, a protective mechanism employed by your subconscious mind to keep your conscious attention on the symptoms and away from those buried dangerous emotions.

My 6-week program has been designed to help you "turn off" these abnormal changes in the body with several mind–body–spirit treatments. In most cases, your symptoms will significantly improve after about forty days—and sometimes earlier.

THREE POWERS BEHIND THE PROGRAM

To get the maximum benefits, you should keep in mind three powers that make the Pain-Free Program successful: time, repetition, and confidence.

THE POWER OF TIME

It will be necessary for you to set aside at least thirty minutes per day to work on this program. Some of my patients put in up to sixty minutes per day, and that's fine. If you can put in more time, you may see even faster results.

I recommend that you do the mind–body–spirit exercises the first thing in the morning, or just before you go to bed. The subconscious mind, which exerts a significant impact on the autonomic nervous system, seems to be the most receptive to input during these times, rather than during a busy, high-pressure day that consumes all your mental attention. Also, your subconscious will tend to be more receptive to processing new healing information when you are more relaxed.

If you want to put in more time—say, up to sixty minutes per day—you can pack your program into a single session. Or you can break it up into two thirty-minute segments, one in the morning and one at night. A lot of times, my Perfectionist personality patients want to do the plan exactly right, and so they'll try to do three or four thirty-minute sessions each day. They usually end up frustrated and irritated because it's almost impossible to find so much time. As a result, I encourage them to *relax*—don't make this program just another pressure in your life. But whatever your choice, *you must make a commitment to put in at least thirty minutes per day*. Without this minimum, you can't expect the best results.

THE POWER OF REPETITION

As you proceed with the program, try not to skip steps. Repetition is critical: It establishes a neuronal connection between your conscious mind and your subconscious mind.

Repetition also moves the truth of what you've learned down into your subconscious mind—a process that causes real changes to occur over time. If you don't see results in a few days, it's easy to lapse into a negative attitude that could tempt you to skip sessions. We have all had feelings like these at one time or another: *Oh, no, it's time for my Pain-Free exercises again! I wish I could get on with my daily business, but . . .*

Try to nip those notions in the bud. Focus immediately on how good it will feel to have your pain go away. Be thankful that you've embarked on a regimen that has the potential to do what all those earlier treatments have failed to do: make you pain-free for life. And remember how powerful repetition can be in forming new habits and creating new "grooves" in your brain and nervous system, which will enable you to influence the activity of your subconscious mind.

In other words, as you move one, two, or three weeks into the program, you'll begin to think more and more in terms of the emotional origin of your pain rather than the old way of thinking about the physical problems. Before long, you'll develop a reflex when you have a muscle twinge, which will cause you to think, *Hey, what emotions are going on down there?* as you recondition your thinking.

It does take time to change your subconscious mind and alter the way it processes the repressed emotions that cause your symptoms.

So employing the power of repetition is important. If you have one of my videos, watch it several times a week (they can be obtained at my Web site, www.BradyInstitute.com). To further engage the power of repetition, read sections of this book over and over (especially chapters 3, 4, and 5). And by all means work on the program assignments every day.

While some chronic pain patients experience pain relief within just two or three weeks, the response to the program is not the same for everyone. Some people are cured after one week, but most take about six weeks to experience significant relief of their symptoms.

If after forty days you don't feel any better, you either do not have a mind–body component to your symptoms, or you have not been successful at uncovering a significant level of repressed and dangerous subconscious emotions. In the latter case, you may need to seek help from a psychologist who understands the process of uncovering repressed emotions—and who can help you achieve this goal. Fortunately, though, less than 15 percent of AOS patients need referral to a psychologist. And again, this step should be made in close consultation with your personal physician.

THE POWER OF CONFIDENCE

The more you learn about Autonomic Overload Syndrome and the subconscious mind—and the more you become confident that you have AOS rather than some structural abnormality—the more power you will gain to get rid of your pain.

In effect, gaining confidence in knowing the true cause of your pain blows the cover of the subconscious mind. Before you develop this confidence, the subconscious mind stays busy keeping your conscious thoughts preoccupied with pain. Your subconscious definitely doesn't want you to focus on the volcano of repressed negative emotions that have been building up and threatening to come out!

But as confidence emerges as a result of insight into your AOS diagnosis, you'll begin an exciting path of discovery. You'll be able to peer with fascination rather than fear down into the repressed emotion volcano as you learn to neutralize the ploys of the subconscious mind. Confidence and insight translate into the power to deal successfully with AOS.

For many—but not all—of my patients, an important ingredient in experiencing the kind of insight that fosters such confidence in the mind–body solution to AOS treatment involves what I call their "aha moment."

EMBRACING YOUR AHA MOMENT

Before we move into a discussion of the details of your 6-week program, back off for a moment and take a deep breath. A number of my patients have told me that after listening to my lectures and tapes, which serve as the foundation for the first part of this book—Understanding Your Pain—they think: *Now it's really starting to make sense to me.* Others say, "When I heard you talk and listened to your tapes, I couldn't believe it: You were talking about me."

You may be experiencing this as well—or if you haven't sensed any particular flash of insight yet, you may very well experience it as you move into the actual program. This personal insight is related in part to the fact that you are developing confidence in what Autonomic Overload Syndrome is and how it works. Most important of all, you're sensing how AOS relates to your particular pain, your repressed emotions, and your pain personality. In other words, your perspective on your pain is shifting.

At the same time, you're probably starting to conclude that pills and other therapies you've tried can't provide you with a lasting solution to AOS symptoms. The structural explanations for your pain have not given you a cure or even long-term pain relief. But even though your pain may have been a mystery when you looked at it from a purely body-medicine point of view, now it's making sense from a mind–body–spirit point of view. If you're beginning to think in these terms, you've hit the aha moment—the time when the psychological explanations for AOS symptoms really start registering.

This moment may occur when you're starting to see yourself in the pages of the book. Perhaps you can identify with something in my story or one of the stories of my patients. It may be that you're a classic pain-prone personality, and the descriptions of one or more of those personalities in chapter 5 clicked with you. Or maybe an insight or cure in one of the other patient case studies that you've read resonates deep inside. It may be that your conviction about this program has caught fire as you have learned how the research of various well-regarded scientists and physicians in leading medical journals has supported the principles we're discussing.

So a kind of lightbulb may have turned on in your mind, and you can now see more clearly that what we've been talking about applies directly to *you* and *your pain*. If you've had this aha moment— or at least if you're very intrigued by now with AOS and the potential of a mind–body–spirit program—you're in a good position to move forward.

With these introductory matters in mind, then, let's plunge directly into the 6-week Pain-Free for Life Program.

THE 6-WEEK PAIN-FREE FOR LIFE PROGRAM

There are five distinct steps in the daily Pain-Free for Life Program, which can be summarized this way:

> *Step 1:* Establish a strong mind–body–spirit link—for five minutes per day.

> *Step 2:* Take control over your subconscious mind—for five
> minutes per day.
>
> *Step 3:* Write about your repressed emotions using the
> depth-journaling technique described in chapter 9—
> for twenty minutes per day.
>
> *Step 4:* Spend time in prayer and meditation—for as long
> as you can.
>
> *Step 5:* Resume physical activity—for as long as you like!

In this chapter, we'll review each step. Then, in the next couple of chapters, we'll go into more depth about steps 2 and 3—which focus on pain talk and depth journaling. Here's how each step works:

STEP 1: ESTABLISH A STRONG MIND–BODY–SPIRIT LINK

When you are suffering from Autonomic Overload Syndrome, which is caused by buried dangerous emotions, it's essential at the outset of every Pain-Free session to close your eyes, sit quietly for about five minutes, and *make the mind–body–spirit link* by focusing on this thought:

It's my repressed emotions—not any physical or structural abnormality—that are causing me to have pain symptoms.

As part of this exercise, always keep this guiding principle in the front of your mind:

You must think of your symptoms in terms of your repressed emotions and the psychological origin of your pain—but not in terms of any physical or structural problem.

Making the mind–body–spirit connection involves establishing a mental or intellectual link between your symptoms and your dangerous emotions, which are hiding deep in your subconscious. In other words, every time you begin a Pain-Free session you should make a mental connection affirming that your AOS symptoms are from those buried emotions *only,* and that there's nothing structurally abnormal with you.

This is an extremely important mind-set to establish before you try anything else, because *your symptoms will continue as long as your mind holds on to the belief that you are abnormal structurally.* And you can be sure that your subconscious mind will constantly try to divert your attention from those dangerous, threatening repressed emotions and toward some phony physical reason for the pain. In effect, your pain symptoms are serving the purpose of keeping your rational, conscious thoughts out of your subconscious mind and away from the dangerous repressed emotions. The pain is a trick—a defense mechanism employed by the subconscious mind.

SHUTTING THE DOOR

It is helpful during this first step of the program to think about *shutting the door to the physical explanations of pain.* To do this, spend some time thinking and imagining the following:

You're standing in the kitchen of a house. There are two doors leading out of the kitchen—one goes to the living room, and one goes to the basement. The living room is well lit and easy to see from the kitchen through the open French doors. The living room represents the physical/structural explanations of your pain. In the living room, a loud audio system is playing propaganda over and over and over in a loop. It goes something like this:

"You're not normal . . . no one will ever be able to cure your pain . . . your X-rays guarantee that you'll never be normal . . . you have a lifelong pain sentence . . . you're weak and frail . . . you've got degenerative disks . . ."

For a long time, all you've listened to is these blaring propaganda tapes playing in the living room. You've heard all the physical explanations, diagnoses, and treatments for your symptoms.

Now I want you to imagine yourself *unplugging* the living room tape player and *closing tight* the French doors that separate the living room and kitchen. Shut those doors, lock them, and throw away the key.

Next, turn around and look at the closed kitchen door that goes down to the basement. The basement represents your subconscious mind, which is filled with old, scary-looking boxes (dangerous emotions) that you've thrown down there day after day after day in an effort to keep them hidden from yourself and anyone else who may happen into your nice house. The basement contains the psychological reasons for your pain and symptoms. So *open* the door to the basement (psychologically) and go down the stairs.

As you do, make the mind–body–spirit link we've discussed. Shut the door to the physical explanations and open the door to the psychological/emotional explanations of your AOS pain. Now, after five minutes of these introductory reflections, you're ready to move on to Step 2 of the program.

STEP 2: TAKE CONTROL OVER YOUR SUBCONSCIOUS MIND

In this step, you are going to use two different mind–body techniques to reverse your subconscious mind's overactivation of your autonomic nervous system. But first, let me introduce you to the science and specifics of practical mind–body techniques—since for many of us they may at first seem unorthodox, to say the least.

Over the past twenty years, researchers have demonstrated that the mind and the body are intimately interconnected—more than we ever realized. Mental exercises have been shown to improve body function in many arenas—including medicine and sports.

In the 1970s, Dr. Herbert Benson at Harvard Medical School

discovered the relaxation response by observing advanced meditators who could use repetitive mental techniques to influence bodily functions previously believed to be beyond the control of the mind. With the mind–body technique of meditation, they could reduce their heart rates, blood pressure, and surface (not core) body temperature. Benson went on to show that the techniques used were not limited to any religious or philosophical tradition and, in fact, could be replicated without any religious trappings whatsoever. In other words, they involve innate capacities shared by all human beings.

In related research, Dr. Jon Kabat-Zinn at the University of Massachusetts Medical Center has used a mind–body technique called mindfulness meditation to help improve skin conditions, pain, surgical outcomes, and chronic illness. He has employed this technique to reduce stress and its effects on the body.

Biofeedback is another popular mind–body technique that has been around for years. Patients, hooked up to instruments that register various brain waves, learn to control and relax body systems with their thoughts—including heart rate, muscle tension, body temperature, and breathing patterns. Biofeedback has been successful in reducing stress, averting headaches, and helping muscle tightness, to list just a few of the benefits.

In the arena of sports, we have also learned a lot about mind–body techniques, which athletes use to enhance performance but can also be applied to AOS pain. Olympic athletes frequently use biofeedback and other mind–body techniques to achieve peak performance. During the 1996 Summer Olympic Games in Atlanta, at least twenty sports psychology consultants worked with Olympic athletes, who employed a variety of mind–body techniques to improve their performance, including:

- ❖ **Imagery.** Mentally rehearsing the performance.
- ❖ **Concentration training.** Learning to tune out distractions.

- ◆ **Relaxation.** Using various mind–body methods and breathing exercises to relax muscles for peak performance.
- ◆ **Visualization.** Mentally "seeing" themselves achieve a particular goal.

Visualization creates a mental picture using the imagination and can influence the mind and muscles in a way that helps athletes get into the proverbial "zone"—and, they hope, to the gold-medal platform.

In the field of professional golf, up to one-third of all PGA Tour members use mind–body techniques, including mental imagery and visualization. Sports psychologists teach pro golfers to visualize themselves striking the ball; to picture the ball in flight; and to see in their mind's eye the exact place where the ball should land.

For example, Davis Love III, one of the top PGA golfers, will take a couple of practice swings before he strikes the ball. After his practice swings, he pauses for a few seconds—visualizing the shot. With repetition and training, such golfers create mental images in their minds that influence the firing of small muscles in their hands and arms. This practice helps them strike the little white ball consistently and putt straight under extreme pressure—right into the final hole on the eighteenth green of the Masters.

In the Pain-Free for Life Program, it's time now for *you*, as part of Step 2, to spend five minutes using two mind–body techniques: pain talk and mental imagery. Both will help change your subconscious mind's overstimulation of the autonomic nervous system. In the process, your autonomic system will turn down, and your symptoms will begin to improve.

A BRIEF INTRODUCTION TO PAIN TALK

To *talk* to your subconscious mind will probably feel a little silly at first—at least it did for me. This mind–body technique involves using your conscious mind to take control over your subconscious mind through speech and thoughts. Up to this point, you've been controlled by your subconscious mind. It produces physical symptoms when it wants, where it wants—and with the intensity it decides. You've been a helpless victim as this is going on, fooled into thinking you're weak and abnormal. But your conscious mind is stronger than your subconscious mind! And you're about to find out how much stronger as you begin taking over operation of your subconscious.

In your pain talk, you might say, "I'm normal! There's nothing physical wrong with me. So stop the pain!"

The main idea is to *talk sternly to your subconscious mind*. As you talk, feel free to *demand* that your subconscious stop your pain—be aggressive! At the same time, keep on repeating to your subconscious that you're normal, and that you won't be tricked:

"My back is normal, I've got bad emotions, not AOS. I'm going to pull those emotions to the surface and think about them. So stop that pain *now*! Okay, subconscious, what emotions are you still trying to hide?"

A friend of mine, a physician in her midforties, once suffered from several AOS symptoms, including chronic headaches, fibromyalgia, and irritable bowel syndrome. Her favorite line, whenever she begins to get any AOS symptoms, is this: "Okay, you can't fool me! What are you trying to hide? I'm going to find out, so stop the pain *now*."

You can talk to yourself silently or out loud. Of course, you may want to be a little careful where you are if you decide to shout. As I mentioned in chapter 2, once while I was on a busy driving range hitting golf balls, I was commanding my subconscious mind to "stop this back spasm right now!" I was rather loud, and when I realized what I had said, it was too late: About ten people had already stopped swinging and were staring directly my way! In any event, it's not the volume that matters; it's the force and conviction with which you confront your subconscious, your buried emotions, and your pain. (We'll go into more detail about how to develop this very important pain-talk technique in chapter 10.)

A second, extremely important mind–body technique that you will find helpful in this step of the program is the use of your imagination, especially through visualization.

IMAGINING A VICTORY

Imagination is a powerful tool for influencing the subconscious mind and autonomic nervous system. If you hear a noise in your home while alone at night—and if you imagine that the sound might be an intruder—just thinking about the danger will cause your autonomic nervous system to turn *up*, your heart to race, and your muscles to get tight. In the imagining exercise used with the Pain-Free Program, however, you will introduce thoughts into your mind that will turn *down* the autonomic activation.

Now spend a few moments using your imagination to picture your conscious mind controlling and winning the pain war against your pain-producing subconscious mind. Here are a few suggestions.

THE COMPUTER SCREEN

I received a thank-you note from a fifty-year-old woman, Christine, who had suffered with fibromyalgia muscle pain for more than twenty years. She wrote:

> *Fibromyalgia felt like the flu: muscle aches, foggy-headed, inability to think straight, confusion. I would often lose my train of thought. Also, I would get periodic migraine headaches and irritable bowel syndrome.*
>
> *I almost always had a constant tension headache and tightness in my neck and shoulders right between my shoulder blades. What I first started doing to get better was convincing myself that the problem wasn't physical—that it was emotional pain I*

was feeling. I would talk to myself, telling myself that this is not physical pain; this is emotional pain.

Also, as I talked out loud, I would visualize—by creating an image in my mind of a computer screen full of words that were my pain symptoms. You know the SCROLL DOWN button? Well, I would imagine that I scrolled down and highlighted all the pain words on the screen—and one by one I would press the DELETE button. Then I would just expect the pain to disappear. And it did *disappear. Sometimes, when the back pains got better, I would start getting a headache, and then shoulder and neck pain. It would seem as though I was chasing the pain all over my body initially, but it finally gave up—and I won!*

THE WARRIOR

Another image that my patients have used successfully involves imagining that you're in a gladiator-type battle with your pain. Representing your conscious mind, you see yourself as stronger than your subconscious mind—the enemy that is constantly creating pain in order to "protect" you, or so it says. But you know your subconscious is working against your best interests. (You might alter this imagery to see your subconscious mind as an invader or robber, or as playing some other threatening role.)

Again, you pull your pain talk into this warrior scenario. Repeat to yourself, "I'm normal and exceptionally strong, and I *will* win this battle. Subconscious, stop the pain now!"

At this point, picture yourself actually knocking down the heavily armed opponent and shoving it into a subordinate role in your life. Now, with your conscious thoughts, you see yourself taking control of your emotions and your pain. You refuse to let your subconscious mind control you or cause pain in your life. Your conscious mind is stronger than the subconscious mind!

As a variation on this theme, you might want to imagine yourself as a great boxer. Close your eyes, relax, and think of a heavyweight boxing match. You're in the white trunks—the up-and-coming contender Mr. Conscious Mind. You're huge and strong and powerful.

Now picture your opponent wearing black trunks—he's the pain-producing champ, Subconscious Mind. For the first eight rounds he's been pounding you pretty well; but now, like Sylvester Stallone in *Rocky*, you're starting to win the fight. Imagine yourself pounding your opponent time after time—and finally winning control. Conscious Mind is in control and the clear new champion.

While you're immersed in this image, it will be helpful to think or say out loud: "Stop the pain! I'm going to win this battle—you have no chance. So stop the pain!"

PICTURING CHANGES IN YOUR BODY

Finally, after you imagine your conscious mind defeating and subjugating your subconscious mind, picture mentally your muscles relaxing and your blood vessels dilating. Imagine the autonomic nervous system speedometer, which has been at a hundred miles per hour, turning down to thirty.

Oxygen-rich blood now begins to flow to your hurting muscles and tendons and nerves. Also, the neuropeptides and neurotransmitters of well-being, such as endorphins and dopamine, which were previously dammed up by stress, are now washing over your muscles, nerves, and tendons, healing and helping them.

By now you've started clearing some fairly strong brain paths from your conscious mind into your subconscious mind. With repetition, you're on your way to a life without AOS pain! Even at this early stage, you may feel your pain beginning to fade. In any event, your time is up, and you move on to the third phase of the program.

STEP 3: WRITE ABOUT YOUR EMOTIONS

All steps in the Pain-Free for Life Program are important, but regular, in-depth journal writing is essential! Your goal should be to spend at least twenty minutes getting your hidden, repressed emotions *out* of your subconscious and *up* to a conscious level. The best way to achieve this result is to record every step of your emotion-discovering journey on paper.

Other ways of describing this process include depth journaling or authoring a personal pain journal—which is exactly what you'll be doing. In other words, you are going to write your own pain story by processing on paper those unprocessed emotions that are causing your pain.

As we saw in previous chapters, Dr. Candace Pert, the neuropeptide researcher, talks about emotions being molecules. In fact, she helped discover the receptor for the molecule of happiness—the endorphin molecule. There is also evidence for real molecules of anger and irritation and fear and guilt.

These dangerous molecules have been stored in boxes deep in your subconscious mind, where they serve to overactivate your autonomic nervous system. The molecules last for years and years unless they're processed (think of a food processor grinding up and destroying the emotions). With this step of journaling out your emotions, you will actually bring these molecules out of the boxes and start processing them—by thinking about them consciously. In this way, you'll neutralize their negative effects on your body.

In this illustration, you redirect the focus of your mind's eye, which used to be focused *up* on the physical pain and symptoms (figure F). Now, however, you look *down* into the subconscious mind (figure G). Of course, you will never be able to think of everything your subconscious has buried or stuffed over your lifetime. But you *will* be able to remember and process many of the danger-

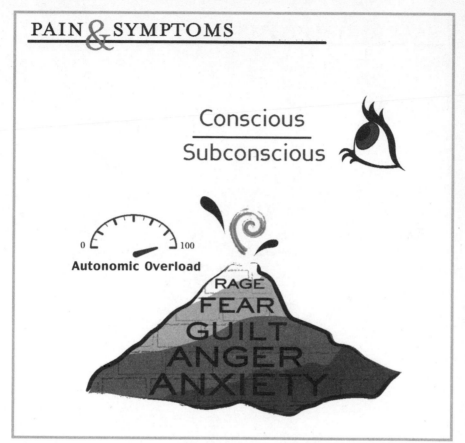

PAIN & SYMPTOMS

Conscious
Subconscious

0 ⌐ 100
Autonomic Overload

RAGE
FEAR
GUILT
ANGER
ANXIETY

Figure F

ous emotions that you're currently unaware of—and that will be enough to stop the pain of AOS.

You can think of this phase of the program as a type of house-keeping, similar to what happened with the kitchen/living room/basement analogy we've already discussed. So as you journal, you'll go down into the basement where all the dangerous, threatening emotions have been thrown and stuffed for years. You'll open up the old boxes and carry them to the first floor, where they can have no harmful effects on your physical body or autonomic nervous system.

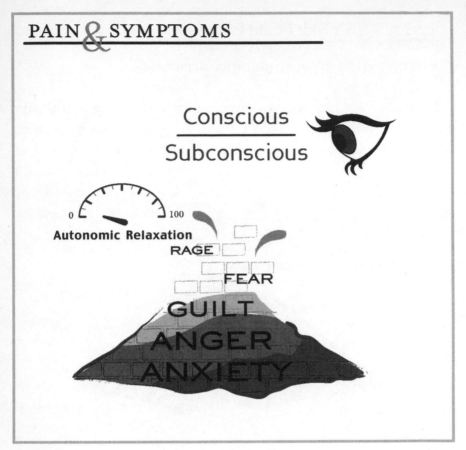

Figure G

When these subconscious thoughts become conscious (when you get them *out* of the basement and are fully aware of them, as in figure G) and they're on your journal paper, your autonomic nervous system will tend to slow down and your muscles will relax more. Then the way will be cleared for your pain symptoms to go away.

What's the best technique for writing your personal pain journal? You can journal a number of ways. As we mentioned in chapter 5 in our discussion of pain-prone personalities, one of the more successful ways to organize your thoughts is to divide the emotions you're going to explore into three categories:

- Emotions from the past.
- Emotions from current circumstances.
- Emotions from your pain-prone personality.

In chapter 9, which focuses in more depth on your personal pain journal, I'll walk you through some illustrations showing how to ask yourself specific questions that will help you explore each of these categories. Also, I'll suggest some types of questions that will help get you started on the right path. But before we go into that kind of detail, it's important to understand some of the basic philosophy and guidelines behind depth journaling.

DO I HAVE TO WRITE?

Sometimes one of my patients will have a tremor or some physical disability that makes it impossible to write. Or sometimes I'll have a patient who says, "Doc, I *hate* to write . . . can't I do this some other way?"

Even though it's important to write out these emotions, you can also talk them out with the help of a trusted friend. Of course, it may not be easy to find a friend who is a great listener and also has twenty minutes every day to work with you. But if this is the route you choose, do the best you can!

REMEMBER THAT DANGEROUS EMOTIONS ARE TRICKY!

When you begin to journal, it may take some time to get to the powerful emotions—after all, you've hidden them fairly successfully. Be especially careful to concentrate on those dangerous emotions that we introduced in chapter 5: anger, fear, guilt, anxiety, and shame.

Also, remember from chapter 5 that these dangerous emotions have ways of hiding in other guises and under other aliases. Anger can look like disappointment, frustration, irritation, or annoyance—though sometimes it becomes recognizable in its strongest form, rage. Fear may show up as worry, uncertainty, hesitancy, or a lack of confidence. Anxiety may hide under the names *nervous* or *upset* or *worried*. Shame often looks like embarrassment or guilt. Whatever name you choose, always start journaling with the least threatening form of the word, and work your way up from there.

You'll recall from my own story that after a few days of journaling for the first time, I only had a couple pages of stuff. I was looking for anger—but I didn't think of myself as an angry person. So the emotion was able to hide pretty well in my subconscious.

But then I decided to start thinking about my past and present circumstances and personality in terms of what "irritated" me. *Wow*—now I had found a gold mine! The word *irritation* was much more acceptable to me at that time. Fast-forward a couple months: I'm at the breakfast table with my wife, and I tell her, "Honey, I can't believe I'm saying this, but I think I'm angry at just about everyone I've ever met . . . most of the time!"

So be ready to take it slow with the depth-journaling process. If you keep at it, you'll get to the dangerous emotions after a while!

STEP 4: SPEND TIME IN PRAYER AND MEDITATION

As we discussed in chapter 6, hundreds of studies in recent years have shown tremendous health benefits when you have an active and rewarding spiritual life. Regular prayer and meditation are the hallmarks of a healthy spiritual life.

But let me emphasize that this fourth phase of the program is *completely optional*. That's one reason why I haven't suggested a time limit for prayer or meditation. Some individuals may want to spend a long time in this spiritual exercise. But I also work with people who don't believe in the spiritual dimension or don't want to include it as part of their Pain-Free for Life Program. In fact, I have many patients who have succeeded in achieving pain-free lives using only mind–body strategies, rather than a mind–body–*spirit* approach.

Still, if you recognize that you have a spiritual side, you will find that your personality, your ability to handle stress, and the quantity of strong negative emotions you experience can be directly affected by your level of spiritual health. So I always hold out Step 4 as a wonderful, if optional, possibility for my AOS patients.

A MEDITATION EXERCISE

No matter where you are in your spiritual journey, from *never-started* to *I'm-a-pastor-of-a-church,* you can experience wonderful benefits in your body, mind, and spirit with the regular practice of prayer and meditation.

If you're new at this meditation thing, don't worry. Actually, we *all* meditate throughout every day—even though we may not be aware of it.

I often ask my patients who are relatively inexperienced in meditation, "What do you think about when you're not thinking about anything?" Or, "What does your mind drift to when it's not focused on a task?"

These are just another way of asking, "What is your mind meditating on?"

In this exercise, I want you to begin by asking yourself that same question: *What do I think about during the day when I'm not thinking about anything?*

You may discover that your mind frequently drifts with worry and anxiety about your future. You might dwell on such topics as where you'll work next year, whom you'll marry, or how your children will fare as they grow older. You may also meditate about what you *should* do, or *could* do—compiling long mental lists of things that silently add to the pressure in your life.

You could be the type of person who thinks a lot about whether people like you or not. Your silent thoughts might include: *I hope I didn't offend her . . . I think she read me the wrong way when I said that . . . I'm afraid he's upset with me.* Or you may meditate many times on things that have gone wrong and people who have let you down. Your mind rehearses why *they're* wrong and *you're* right. Whatever the content, it's helpful to uncover the silent thoughts that go through your mind just below the level of full consciousness. This process may provide you with some clues about what you've been burying for years deep in your subconscious.

Now, as the next step in this meditative exercise, I want you to begin to *direct* your thoughts a little more toward anything in your life that is good, lovely, beautiful, hopeful, or joyful. I call this step directed meditation. Maybe you want to think about something you know for certain is wonderful and true, such as *God is in control,* or *God loves me just as I am,* or *My kids are awesome, they love just being with me.* You may want to direct your thoughts to a short, positive Scripture verse, such as "God is love."

Next, focus on your blessings—the things you have to be thankful for. Since you meditate throughout the day, not just for the few minutes that may be involved in this fourth step, resolve to think about these things as often as you can throughout the rest of this day.

THE PLACE OF PRAYER

Finally, if you feel comfortable doing it, take a few minutes at the end of your session to pray. Prayer is simply talking honestly and openly to God. Maybe you're angry with God, or you feel completely alone, or you're not sure God exists. Any of those thoughts is perfectly okay.

God may seem cold to you, like an impersonal and harsh judge. A lot of my patients, even those who are deeply spiritual, say that their view of God is that of an irritated father—and they're just waiting for the other shoe to drop. It's okay for you to feel that way, too. As you pray, just say whatever is on your mind; most important, be honest with your feelings. Your utterance may be only a few words of thanks or praise, or it may be a tirade full of anger or sorrow that you want to share with God.

Now shift your prayers to your pain:

- Talk to God freely about the pain you're feeling.
- Ask him to direct your path out of the pain—and toward him.
- Talk to God about the emotions you're beginning to find inside yourself, now that you're actually starting on your 6-week program.

To sum up, no matter where you are on your spiritual journey, take a couple of minutes to talk to God about where you are, what you're thinking, and where you want to be in relationship to him. And always be aware that it's quite appropriate to put your pain on the agenda during your encounters with him.

STEP 5: RESUME PHYSICAL ACTIVITY

Most people suffering from chronic pain give up an active physical life. Favorite sports are often the first thing to go: I quit playing golf because I believed the twisting might hurt my "bad back." I also gave up lifting weights because my back would sometimes hurt worse after a workout. Of course, I had been fooled into this inactivity by my subconscious brain and the fear that I might make things worse. Perhaps you're in a similar situation with your favorite sport or activity.

Many people wrestling with AOS pain give up things they once enjoyed: exercise, taking long trips in a car, going to the movies, playing tennis, or dancing, to name a few. They may also elect not to engage in an active sex life—because they're afraid their "bad back" will go out. Or they refuse to bend over to pick up items off the floor, or tend to their garden, or do chores around the house, again because of the worry about straining their back or pushing themselves too much.

Now, in the final step of this program, you must resume those physical activities you've stopped. Of course, if your physician was the one to tell you to stop—please check with him or her *before* you restart.

When you have AOS pain during physical activity, always remember that your physical body is *normal*. Your pain is caused by your emotions, and there's no reason your physical body can't do those things you once enjoyed. In short, I want you to forget your fears and hesitations. Recall that you have already gone through a battery of tests to ensure that you don't have any structural emergencies going on. (Or at least you *should* have gone through those tests. If you haven't, put down this book right now and make an appointment with your doctor for a thorough physical exam!)

Timing is critical when you decide to become active again. I ask most patients to wait until they are three to four weeks into the Pain-Free for Life Program before they take up those activities that they're afraid of. Of course, you could begin your workouts on the very first day—but I prefer that you begin to feel better and gain confidence in the program before you attack the gym again.

Confidence is *huge* in the process of AOS recovery—and your subconscious mind knows it. So when you begin to engage in those activities and exercises you once did, you can expect the subconscious to *turn up your symptoms* in a last-ditch effort to keep you away from the dangerous emotions you've started to explore— emotions that the subconscious is trying so hard to protect. Be ready to fight with your subconscious mind!

Having said this, I want to remind you that if you develop any *new* symptoms that haven't been evaluated yet by your physician— you'll need to check them out.

So in three or four weeks you should begin to move gradually back toward your former level of activity, with the assurance that when you finally put your emotional house in order, you'll be able to return to your old level of activity. Obviously, you'll have to take some time getting back in shape and returning to the level of fitness and skill that you enjoyed before the pain—before your subconscious robbed you of the joy and fun you had with a more active life. But that will be relatively easy after the battles you have been through with your subconscious and your most dangerous emotions.

So finally you have launched your Pain-Free for Life Program. Resolve immediately to spend thirty minutes every day, beginning at a *specific* time, evening or morning. Take each of the above steps in order and repeat these steps every day for forty days.

Now you're on your way to becoming pain-free and enjoying *life*! But to increase your skill in these mind–body–spirit techniques still further—and to boost your confidence in employing them to banish your pain—the following chapters have been designed to make you a real Pain-Free for Life expert. In particular, you're about to learn probably all you'll ever need to know about depth journaling and pain talk.

DEPTH
JOURNALING

It's no secret: Getting dangerous emotions out of your mind and spirit, and onto a piece of paper, has amazing health benefits. Consider this rather startling research report:

In 1999, the *Journal of the American Medical Association* (*JAMA*) printed a study done at the State University of New York at Stony Brook involving 112 patients who suffered from rheumatoid arthritis and asthma.[1] Between 1996 and 1997, these 112 patients were divided up into randomized controlled groups.

Seventy-one of them (thirty-nine with asthma and thirty-two with rheumatoid arthritis) were asked to write about the most stressful event in their lives. The remaining forty-one were asked to write about "emotionally neutral" topics such as their daily plans (as you might do in a diary). They all were instructed to write for twenty minutes each day *for only three consecutive days*. Each patient was reexamined at intervals of two weeks, two months, and four months after the three-day journal-writing exercise.

The researchers found that 47 percent of the group that wrote about very stressful experiences had substantial improvement in their symptoms. Of those who wrote about emotionally neutral topics, 24 percent improved, and 21 percent got worse.

To put this another way, the people in this study only did sixty *total* minutes of journal writing—and they were only asked to write about *one* stressful event in their life—yet almost *half* of them had significant improvement of their symptoms.

Now consider your situation. Imagine what would happen if you journaled twenty minutes a day for forty days, and as a result you journaled out many of those toxic emotions that lie resting in the vault of your subconscious mind. Clearly, this sort of depth journaling could have amazing health benefits—including the potential of making you pain-free!

Of course, the study was no surprise to me or to hundreds of patients who have been through the Brady Institute's Pain-Free for Life Program. My patients have understood for years that depth journaling is a critical piece of the recovery plan for those who suffer from symptoms of Autonomic Overload Syndrome. Barbara is just one of many who has been freed from chronic pain by practicing this very thing.

BARBARA WRITES HER WAY OUT OF PAIN

For years, Barbara had been living with back and leg pain, which had started just after she was in a car accident. She had been hit from behind and was diagnosed at the outset with bursitis, but her diagnosis was later changed to sciatic nerve pain (or sciatica). Over the next few years, she consulted with about half a dozen different physicians. She had a few micro surgeries that didn't help for long, and her specialist finally told her: "You may never get completely better, and the older you get, the worse pain you can expect."

"I would get a sharp shooting pain down my bottom and the back of my leg," she said, "sometimes it felt like a bad toothache. I stopped going to movies, which was one of the favorite things my family likes to do together. But I was afraid of taking pain pills: I didn't want to get stuck on them. So I just quit going to events that required me to sit for any extended period."

Desperate for help, Barbara tried several pain clinic programs and underwent multiple injections into her lower back, with no results. "The last time, I think I counted sixty-six injections, but I was still left with a burning, throbbing pain all the time," she said.

Then Barbara turned to acupuncture, but the acupuncturist predicted that it would take "a long time" to see any results. Another specialist said he thought she had a nerve that was stuck between two tendons; he guessed that sitting caused pain in her sciatic nerve. Still another doctor actually advised her to quit her job and walk dogs for a living.

After she had exhausted every medical and quasi-medical avenue she could think of, she found her way to my office. As a result of our preliminary interview and physical exam, I concluded that her sciatic nerve, muscles, and the bones of her spine were all normal for her age. In addition, I saw that she was a clear People-Pleaser personality and that she wasn't comfortable with anger or other strong emotions. Barbara had Autonomic Overload Syndrome. As a result, I expected that she could benefit significantly from our 6-week program.

Before long, Barbara was going through each step of our program daily. In particular, she was finding special insights, as most of our patients do, during the depth-journaling phase. As I initially explained to Barbara, depth journaling is not complicated, but it is very different from keeping a daily diary.

WHAT BARBARA UNDERSTOOD ABOUT DEPTH JOURNALING

Depth journaling is different from writing daily events down in a diary or writing down memories and spiritual insights in a journal.

Instead, it is an in-depth self-analysis and self-discovery exercise that uncovers repressed dangerous emotions.

Think of those buried, subconscious emotions as a kind of onion, which the "author" (AOS patient) must peel off, layer after layer. The longer she peels, the deeper into the onion she'll get. And the deeper she gets, the more emotionally charged she'll find her memories to be. Finally, as she continues to delve deeper and discover more by writing in her journal, her pain will become better.

That's exactly what happened to Barbara.

At first, she conceded, she wasn't sure that writing in a journal would work for her. "But I went home and started writing that very first day, and I kept on trying," she said.

As the centerpiece of Step 3 of the Pain-Free for Life Program, the depth-journaling phase is absolutely essential because it enables you to concentrate over relatively long periods of time (twenty straight minutes) on your inner life and stuffed emotions. Only when you devote time and effort to this exercise can you hope to identify the dangerous and hidden emotions inside and then drag them to the surface. And once you've laid them out on the paper in front of you, their power over you fades because they're no longer in the subconscious mind—driving the autonomic nervous system; they're in the conscious mind at this point, and they have no power to cause pain.

BARBARA'S MIDCOURSE CORRECTION

I suspected that Barbara was having some trouble getting into her journaling, so I called her to follow up. She told me, "I find that I'm always apologizing to myself in the journal for writing down things I think I shouldn't be writing. I feel guilty about the process. Also, when I find a particular emotion, I feel guilty that I had it in the past and buried it."

I smiled to myself because I knew that now she was getting to a good place, and I knew exactly what she was thinking—being somewhat of a People-Pleaser myself. So I said, "What you're feeling—the guilt and anxiety about having those emotions—is exactly what you should expect to be feeling. You want to please people so much that even *writing* about how someone irritates and angers you is almost too much for you. That's exactly why you got pain in the first place: *You can't stand these emotions,* so you reflexively stuff them. But I like what I'm hearing, so keep at it! The more you explore your emotional basement and uncover those destructive emotions, the easier it will get. More important, the more you do it, the closer you'll move toward a pain-free life."

So Barbara kept at it.

BARBARA DIGS IN

As she wrote, she discovered that one of her biggest sources of guilt was her concern over not always being able to please her husband and family. Things only got worse after she developed sciatic nerve pain: "I worried the whole time we went to movies because I knew I wasn't going to be able to sit through the whole thing, and I didn't want to disappoint my family. Then I'd get a little depressed, thinking that I was never going to get better, never going to be able to travel with the family or do other things that I loved to do."

Dinner parties were also hard for her. As long as she was in a place where she could get up and walk around, she was okay. But having to sit for a long time in a crowded restaurant, or being wedged into a dining room with a large group of family and friends, could be excruciating.

Among the things she discovered about herself during her depth journaling was that she was often afraid she was going to hurt someone's feelings; people might not think well of her. To prevent this disturbing emotion, she always resorted to serving others, smiling, and being nice and sweet—even when she didn't feel like it. She sensed she had to put on a facade and hide her true emotions or she would run the risk of exposing herself to others (and herself) as "not really being as nice as I had hoped and pretended."

But the pain made it impossible for her to live up to the expectations she felt others had of her. As she suffered these inner conflicts, she bottled up her emotions, assuming that the least she could do for others was to keep them from knowing how miserable she felt.

"I realized that I was causing myself even more pain by keeping all these worries and frustrations inside and not venting what I really felt," she said. "Also, I was afraid that if I began to discuss my feelings, I might get into an argument. So it was easier just not to say anything at all, but swallow those emotions silently."

On one occasion, while I was talking to Barbara and her husband, she told me proudly about what she considered to be one of the biggest achievements in her life: She had been married for more than twenty years, but she and her husband had engaged in only about three arguments.

I could have let the comment pass, but I decided to take a chance on her emotional strength by responding honestly: "Actually, that's not really an achievement. It sounds very unhealthy to me. All good marriages involve conflicts and arguments—but the art of moving through conflict with forgiveness keeps the marriage strong. Not arguing is one of the ways that you stuff your strongest negative emotions. You push them deep inside, and they have no way to find release—except through your back and sciatic pain."

Over several weeks, she was able to pull many dangerous emotions to the surface and get them on paper in her steadily growing depth journal. When she revealed to me what she was discovering about herself, I explained, "It's like a volcano. Once you start keeping everything inside, the pressure just builds and builds. The only way it can come out is through a massive emotional explosion—like a panic attack or emotional breakdown . . . or through AOS pain and symptoms. But the more you release some of those emotions through your journal writing, the more your pain will subside."

THE DEPTH JOURNAL AS SAFETY VALVE
An especially important principle that I passed on to Barbara was that her depth journal could serve as a kind of safety valve to keep her from emotional outbursts that might hurt or alienate friends or loved ones. She liked that idea!

"When I first started the program, I thought Dr. Brady was going to suggest that I become the kind of person that I couldn't be," she recalled. "In other words, when I first went to his opening lecture on pain, I thought he was going to tell me that if I was really mad about something, I should just blurt it out. I was relieved to see that wasn't what he wanted at all. Instead, he said, 'If you feel like lashing out, write your feelings down in your journal. Then, if you want to—if you just can't stand seeing those feelings there in black and white—throw it away! Burn it! Get rid of it in whatever way you like.'"

THE PROOF IS IN THE JOURNAL
After only about two or three weeks, Barbara really got into the swing of depth journaling. She began to feel quite comfortable searching for her buried dangerous emotions—including guilt, fear, and anger—and writing extensively about them in her journal. She spent only the recommended twenty minutes or so per day with her journaling, but the impact on her pain was dramatic.

By the time she finished the program, her pain had disappeared. Now, she says, "I go to everything and do everything I want. We're leaving for New York in the morning. Also, I'm working more than I was before. I pretty much do everything that I did prior to the accident."

Barbara's commitment to the *entire* Pain-Free for Life Program was essential to her recovery. But there is no doubt that if she had to pick one decisive factor in banishing pain from her life, it would be her commitment to depth journaling.

So what can you learn from Barbara's experience? First, let me mention a few guidelines for writing a successful depth journal. Then I'll lead you step by step through some model questions that should help you find and pull to the surface of your consciousness those repressed dangerous emotions in your own life.

USE YOUR JOURNAL TO DIVIDE THE MOUNTAIN

As you launch your journal, try fixing this image in your mind:

Over time, your dangerous emotions have been stored in the depths of your subconscious mind. Think of these emotions as big rocks—piled on each other day after day and year after year. After a while, the subconscious mind has a full-fledged *mountain* of built-up repressed dangerous emotions driving the autonomic nervous system to produce AOS pain (see figure H).

As mentioned briefly in chapter 8, it's helpful to think of this mountain as being divided into three parts, as shown on page 197, with rocks from the *past*, rocks from your *current circumstances*, and rocks from your *pain-prone personality*.

As you're about to begin your twenty-minute depth-journaling exercise each day, you should first decide which of these three parts of the mountain you're going to think about—and then focus on your chosen rock pile.

YOUR ROCK PILE OF THE PAST

Ever since childhood, you've been adding big dangerous rocks to your subconscious mind. The key is this: *These memories and*

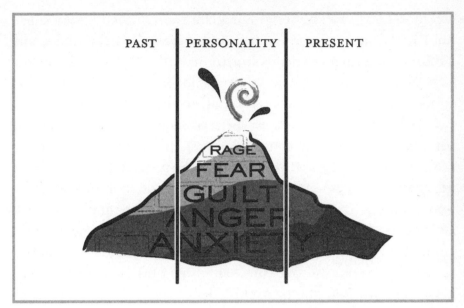

Figure H

events—dangerous emotion rocks—can stay with you the rest of your life.

To use another metaphor, your subconscious mind is also like the hard drive of a computer. You might not see dangerous, emotionally charged memories as one of your visible desktop icons. But sure enough, they're down in the hidden files of your mental computer: You downloaded them a long time ago, and they never left. You haven't looked at them for a while—but now you're about to find them, look at them (on paper), and delete the files.

In the *past* section of your subconscious mountain, you will find all those dangerous, emotion-attached memories that you experienced as a child, a teenager, and so on. You may have suffered major emotional trauma from abuse or neglect or abandonment; if you did, these issues are so huge that you may want to consider getting professional assistance to carry out the boulders.

Many times, AOS patients who have experienced these profound childhood evils will say, "I did suffer child abuse when I was a kid—but I've thought about it and talked to a counselor a few times, and I think I've gotten over it." No, you haven't. This boulder is too large and dangerous; at best you've probably only pulled up a few small rocks from the sides. Go there again and see what you find.

Other major boulders from the past include divorced parents, parental death, verbally abusive parents, absent parents, and even moving around a lot. Of course, this list isn't exhaustive, but you get the idea. These events bring major-league amounts of emotional trauma to children and young adults. Just think of what a child goes through when a parent dies—anger and rage, huge amounts of fear, guilt for any number of reasons, anxiety about the future, and so on. But only small amounts of these emotions ever get expressed. Like the proverbial tip of the iceberg, they stand above a huge mass of ice and rock, a mountain of dangerous emotions.

Other patients tell me that they've had a good childhood; they weren't abused and they grew up with a mom and dad who seemed to love them. In this case, I ask them to focus on two words: *responsibility* and *pressure*.

Of course, every child needs to learn responsibility, but too much responsibility in childhood results in a lot of repressed anger. Kids really need a chance to be kids. Like many of my patients, however, you may have had to take on way too much responsibility when you were younger. Maybe your mom died, and, as the older sister, you had the responsibility of filling in as a caretaker much too soon. Responsibility creates anger in childhood when it's too much, too soon.

Another buzzword that can help you dig up the boulders of your past is *pressure*. Like responsibility, children should not have to carry a lot of pressure on their shoulders. Too much causes frustration and anger.

I find this response to be common in children of preachers and missionaries, or children of parents with a Legalist or Perfectionist personality. These parents often expect their children to behave perfectly and follow all the rules nearly perfectly. It all seems right to the parent, but the child, who smiles and says "yes sir" all the time, is under an inordinate amount of pressure. If you grew up in a house where rules were the main value, you were probably under too much pressure, and, as you depth journal, you're going to find a lot of strong emotions associated with that pressure.

YOUR ROCK PILE OF PRESENT CIRCUMSTANCES

The second rock pile you'll want to explore in your journaling takes you out of the past and into the present. As part of my patient interview, I always ask the question, "What are the three biggest stressors in your entire life?"

Almost always, patients don't even consider the past or the stress associated with their pain-prone personality. They go right toward all the stressful circumstances in their present-day life.

Present-day stressful circumstances generate tons of dangerous emotions. When you think of stress, think of it in terms of the dangerous emotional response it causes in you. Think about the anger and frustration and anxiety associated with that stress. Too much stress can be bad for you; we all know that.

In fact, we've known this since 1967, when researchers Thomas Holmes and Richard Rahe published a "Social Readjustment Rating Scale" in the *Journal of Psychosomatic Research*.[2] Holmes and Rahe thought that if you scored high on this stress scale, you were at risk for developing serious disease and illness. (Clearly, the roots of mind–body research have been around for a while!)

Although the study is about four decades old, it continues to be a helpful tool as we evaluate the current stress in our lives. Of course, when this study was published, stressors didn't include "fear of a terrorist attack," or "my country is in a global war without battle lines," or many other things that might make the list today. Nevertheless, the researchers concluded that if you have a score of 150 or less, you have a 37 percent chance of becoming seriously ill. Between 150 and 300, the risk jumps to 51 percent. Over 300, there is an 80 percent chance of serious illness in the next two years.

The Holmes-Rahe Scale is listed below. But as you go through the questions, use the scale as a kind of checklist to be sure you are covering in your journal writing all the major stressors now in your life. To this end, it may be helpful to keep several thoughts in mind.

First, you'll see that *all change is stressful*—positive and negative. Also, one of the biggest emotion-generating stressors is *not being in control*. So allow the scale to jog your memory about situations where you're currently not in control. Finally, remember that Autonomic Overload Syndrome has nothing to do with stress levels alone. Rather, it has to do with the repressed strong dangerous emotions associated with the stress.

So as you reflect on your major life events during the last twelve months, circle any of the things that pertain to you. Add up the score and see what you find. If you circle a stressor, write beside it any of the dangerous emotions the stress may have caused in your life. Then transfer those notes to your depth journal.

THE HOLMES-RAHE SCALE

STRESSOR	RATING
Death of a spouse	100
Divorce	60
Menopause	60
Separation from living partner	60
Jail term or probation	60
Death of close family member	60
Serious personal injury or illness	45

THE HOLMES-RAHE SCALE (CONT.)

STRESSOR	RATING
Marriage/establish a life partner	45
Fired at work	45
Marital/relationship reconciliation	40
Retirement	40
Change in health of family member	40
Work more than forty hours per week	35
Pregnancy or causing pregnancy	35
Sex difficulties	35
Gain of new family member	35
Business or work role change	35
Change in financial status	35
Death of close friend	30
More arguments with spouse	30
Large loan or mortgage	25
Loan or mortgage foreclosure	25
Sleep less than eight hours per night	25
Change in work responsibility	25
Trouble with children or in-laws	25
Outstanding personal achievement	25
Spouse begins or stops work	25
Begin school or end school	20
Change in living conditions	20
Change in personal habits (diet or the like)	20
Chronic allergies	20
Trouble with boss	20
Change in work hours	20
Moving to new residence	20
Change in schools	20
Change in religious activity	20
Vacation	10
Presently in winter season	10
Minor violation of the law	5

The third rock pile of the mountain is made up of the boulders you've repressed and built up as a result of your pain-prone personality. We won't go into this again here because the salient information you need is contained in chapter 5. But you should read that chapter periodically to remind yourself how just being you can cause lots of strong negative emotions, including anger, every day.

START WRITING!

Now you have a format to begin your depth journaling.

First, you'll think of the part of the mountain that you want to write about today—your past, your current circumstances, or your pain-prone personality (see chapter 5).

Next, you'll pick *one* emotion from the section in chapter 4 on dangerous emotions, and think only about this emotion during your twenty minutes. Try to formulate a few leading questions to get you started.

Here are a few examples:

DAY 1 **THE PAST**	EMOTION: **FEAR**

1. My greatest fear as a child was . . .
2. I used to have lots of nightmares about . . .
3. The thing that scared me the most was . . .
4. When I got scared, I would . . .

DAY 2 **THE PAST**	EMOTION: **SHAME**

1. In my life, I'm most ashamed of . . .
2. My parents would make me feel embarrassed by . . .
3. The thing that embarrassed me the most was . . .

DAY 3 PRESENT CIRCUMSTANCES	EMOTION: ANXIETY

1. The thing that makes me the most nervous is . . .
2. I get anxious when I think about or talk about . . .
3. The worst thing that could happen in my life is . . .

DAY 4 MY PERFECTIONIST PERSONALITY	EMOTION: ANGER

1. The thing that irritates me most about people is . . .
2. Pressure makes me angry. The things that cause me pressure are . . .
3. Responsibility makes me angry. I feel like I'm responsible for . . .
4. I'm the most disappointed in . . .

At the end of this chapter, I'll give you several pages of additional questions that you can use to stimulate your thinking still more. But first, let me share some tips that I've learned from my personal depth journaling as well as from talking to hundreds of AOS patients.

FIVE TIPS FOR DEPTH JOURNALING

These tips are by no means an exhaustive list. You will probably think of others that work well for you. But I've found that these five will get most people started successfully with their journals.

TIP 1: KEEP TRACK OF YOUR PAIN INTENSITY

Many patients find it helpful to record every day—and perhaps several times during the course of a day—how their pain feels on a scale of one to ten, with one being no pain and ten being unbearable pain. I found it very encouraging to look back in my journal, see a bunch of eights and nines, and realize how much better I had gotten. You may not believe it now, but you will quickly forget what pain is like once you're pain-free.

Also, recording the intensity of your pain helps you begin to see the connection between your emotions and your physical symptoms. For a while, you won't understand why one day you're a five, and the next you're a seven. Later on, you'll begin to recognize the hidden forces behind this—the pressures and stresses and repressed emotions associated directly with the intensity of your pain.

In any case, I believe that in order to monitor how you're doing with your pain—and what mind–body–spirit treatments seem to work best—it will be helpful to maintain some sort of ongoing pain intensity record.

TIP 2: FOCUS ON YOUR INNER LIFE— NOT ON YOUR DAILY SCHEDULE

There may be a temptation as you depth journal to slip into a "Dear Diary" mode, with the primary emphasis on people you meet or things you do during the day.

While outside events and encounters with people may be relevant in your journaling, it's important always to keep your eye on the ball: Your main objective is to write an *emotional* autobiography. Also, the process is called *depth journaling* to differentiate it from a random list of events and people. Of course, when you search your past, you'll want to remember and relive certain events; but always remember to go for the dangerous emotions related to that event, not just for the event itself.

For example, if you had an alcoholic father who constantly embarrassed you in front of your friends or abused you or other members of your family, you undoubtedly felt anger and shame when you were around him. It's likely that you repressed most of those dangerous emotions—if you expressed them openly, you were likely to get whacked or shamed even more. In such a case, you would obviously include references to your father and other individuals and to particular events that have become riveted in your memory. But the main focus should not be on the events or the people, but the emotions they triggered in you.

TIP 3: GO DEEPER AND DEEPER

As mentioned earlier, writing an effective depth journal may be somewhat like peeling an onion. After you discover the edge of one layer and peel it back, you find another, even more pungent layer. Then, repeating the process, you discover a layer that is smellier still.

In this same vein, the chances are that on your first try, you'll just scratch the surface of your fear, your anger, or your shame. For that matter, on your initial run-through, you may not identify *any* dangerous emotions inside yourself. But if you keep on writing—almost as though you're operating with a "writer's automatic pilot" driving you—you'll soon see insights and facts pop up on paper that you never thought about before.

But this sequence of events, which can lead you to your real mother lode of pain-causing emotions, may never begin to unfold unless you write, and then write some more.

TIP 4: WRITE LONG AND FREELY

Good writing is often said to be tight and succinct, with no wasted words. But in depth journaling, you're engaged in writing a first draft, not priceless prose for posterity. You're free-thinking, not writing for a college term paper. Also, don't worry about grammar, spelling, or penmanship. You're free to make mistakes—please don't put yourself under any more pressure trying to write everything perfectly.

Also, it's been said that journaling is "baring your heart on paper." Depth journaling is a very private and personal matter—you're exploring the recesses of your heart. You might laugh or cry when you're writing. When you're done with a page, you're free to save it for reflection later on. Or you're free to tear it out and rip it up.

Sometimes I have used visualization techniques when I've journaled. I might think of the toxic emotion flowing from my back, out my arm, and through my pen onto the paper. When it was finally all out—I was free.

So don't worry about repeating yourself or saying things the wrong way or writing with brevity. The more you write, the more likely it will be that somewhere in that sea of words you'll record important facts and insights that will help you expose the hidden emotions responsible for your AOS pain and symptoms.

TIP 5: ALWAYS CARRY AROUND A WRITING PAD

Most people seem to prefer the comfort of using an old-fashioned paper journal for their entries. Somehow, settling down in a quiet place with a pen and a diary-type journal engenders a relaxed focus that is lacking with other techniques. But increasingly, patients who regularly write on computers are turning to electronic devices— and there's certainly nothing wrong with this approach.

Whatever you use, however, I emphasize the importance of always being ready to respond when a flash of insight about your pain or your buried emotional life comes to mind. If you don't capture these fleeting thoughts when they occur, you may lose them again quickly. So always try to arm yourself with a writing pad when you're out and about—as does one of my patients, whom I'll call Paul.

Paul suffered from back pain that clocked in regularly at a nine or ten on my pain scale. As with Barbara, his pain began with a car accident. But he then exacerbated it while riding on his motorcycle.

"I couldn't exercise, ride my motorcycle, pick up anything— there was virtually nothing I could do that I wanted to do," he said. "The only thing I wanted to do anymore was to make myself comfortable!"

Diagnostic tests had revealed that he had five herniated disks. But as you already know—and as Paul learned—herniated disks don't necessarily translate into pain. Paul's pain had resulted in a severely restricted lifestyle.

"It got so bad that I didn't enjoy doing anything—going out to dinner, just living," he said. "When you have constant pain, everything else is put on hold and becomes secondary."

I've discovered that Paul's evaluation of the impact of chronic pain on daily life applies to every one of my patients: They can't carry on a productive social life, love life, work life, spiritual life, or exercise life. In his case, doctors initially recommended a back operation. They also instructed him to suspend all unessential activity—in effect, to do nothing—because anything he did seemed to increase his pain.

But Paul didn't like the idea of an operation, and so, as a last resort, he came to me. He immediately latched onto the principles of our program, or—as he says—"I believed it!"

In particular, he focused on depth journaling. The technique worked so well in helping him delve into his subconscious and pull out dangerous pain-causing emotions that he began to focus on his writing more than anything else.

"I always carry a pad with me," he said, referring to the frequent business trips he takes. "If I'm on the road on the way to see a customer, I may start feeling tight. So I'll pull off the road and write down what's really bothering me. If I park on the side of the road and write for five minutes, the pain and discomfort go away. Then I can go on about the rest of my day."

What's Paul's current pain status? "Right now, I feel great—though people I talk to about this have a hard time believing it. But I tell them I'm living proof because now I'm doing anything I want to do. I've got a home up in the woods, where I go to chop wood. And I can ride my motorcycle anywhere I like—without a bit of pain."

By actually stopping and dealing with his pain at the first inkling that it was about to return, Paul developed a pain-free maintenance practice that has continued to work for him in his recovery. And the key to his success has been that simple little pad that he carries with him everywhere he goes.

These few basic tips should help you get started with your depth journal. But even after you get settled in your chair and start writing, you may find you are blocked as you try to identify and deal with repressed feelings and emotions. To help break the logjam, here are some questions that I have developed.

QUESTIONS TO BREAK YOUR EMOTIONAL LOGJAMS

If you need help asking yourself questions during your journaling time, the questions below may jog your repressed memories and emotions. But don't simply answer them quickly with a yes or no. Instead, the point is to think for a while, let your ruminations dig up some stuffed emotions—and get them out on the journal pages!

QUESTIONS ABOUT YOUR PAST
1. What was life like with your father (or mother)?
2. When did he encourage you?
3. What was family discipline like?
4. Was he an alcoholic? Did he have another addiction?
5. Did he embarrass you in front of others? How?
6. Did you feel responsible for taking care of your family or siblings?
7. What pressure did you feel when you were around your family?

8. What was life like: relaxed, full of expectations, full of pressure?
9. What were the unwritten rules in your family?
10. What were your parents' expectations of you?
11. Did you have to be nice and good . . . or be right and punctual and correct?
12. If you were involved in religion, did it free you up, or load you down with rules and regulations?
13. What did you grow up thinking about God?
14. Do you feel like you have a personal relationship with God?
15. Do you feel a lot of guilt or anger when talking about religion?
16. Did your parents allow you to be adventurous, or did you have to be "safe"?
17. What's the saddest thing you remember about your childhood?
18. What's the happiest memory of your childhood?
19. What were the three biggest pressures you faced growing up? Do you still feel them?
20. Did your mother or father die when you were growing up? What was that like?
21. Were you the popular kid? Did you feel you had to be a phony? Was there a lot of pressure?
22. Were you the unpopular or unrecognized kid? How did it feel?
23. How did you show anger growing up?
24. What was your biggest fear as a kid?
25. What are you most ashamed of?
26. What are you most guilty about?
27. Were your parents divorced? Write out how you felt the day you found out.

28. Did you think it was your fault? Do your parents know how much the divorce hurt you?
29. Did your parents fight a lot? What was that like? How did you feel when they fought?

QUESTIONS ABOUT YOUR CURRENT CIRCUMSTANCES

1. What are the three biggest pressures you feel now?
2. Exactly how do you behave when you're stressed out, angry, or afraid?
3. What is the greatest weight on your shoulders right now? Describe it in detail.
4. Do you laugh a lot? Why, or why not?
5. Describe your marriage and your other close relationships. What's most disappointing? What's most frustrating?
6. Describe your financial worries.
7. What makes you feel out of control?
8. Is your life disappointing to you? Explain.
9. How do you and your spouse have disagreements? Do you avoid them?
10. Do you hate conflict? Why?
11. What pressure does your spouse put on you?
12. What pressure do *you* put on yourself?
13. What are your three biggest responsibilities?
14. What rules do you operate by?
15. What things do people do that anger you the most? What are your pet peeves?
16. What's the most restful thing that you can imagine?
17. What especially riles you up?
18. Do you ever think about dying? Are you afraid to even talk about death? Why?
19. What is your biggest personal failure in the past two years? The past five years? The past ten years? In your life?

20. How is your relationship with your children? Do you think you should be a better father or mother?
21. Make a list of shoulds and oughts in your life. For example: "I should do _____. I should not _____." Was the list easy to make? How do all these things make you feel?
22. When is the last time you felt really free and relaxed?
23. Are you currently doing something that you know you shouldn't? How do you feel after you've done it? How would you feel if you got caught?
24. What do you dream about?
25. What's the biggest fear you have?
26. When your mind wanders, what do you think about?
27. What things preoccupy your mind: finances, your weight, death, fear of war, or something else? Write about them.
28. What is the thing that you are most ashamed of in your life?
29. Is there anything you don't want anyone to know about you?
30. What things make you feel guilty?

QUESTIONS RELATED TO YOUR PAIN PERSONALITY

For some ideas in this area, it will be helpful again for you to look back over the descriptions, mottoes, and questions in chapter 5, Understanding Your Pain-Prone Personality. To give you an idea about how you might draft a series of questions tailored specifically to your particular pain-prone personality, here are a couple of models, based on what you've already learned about the Perfectionist and People-Pleaser personalities:

The Perfectionist

1. Make a list of three things you didn't do right in the past week.
2. What expectations do you put on yourself?

3. What are your expectations of others?
4. What three things anger you most about yourself?
5. What things anger you most about others?
6. What pressures do you put on yourself?
7. How do you feel when you don't do something well?
8. What disappoints you the most?
9. How do people make you angry most often?

The People-Pleaser

1. Are relationships hard for you? Are you involved in much relational conflict?
2. Are you angry at yourself about this?
3. What pressure do you feel?
4. What would happen if you told everyone what you really think about them?
5. Choose three people you are close to, and write out what you really think about them.
6. How do you sacrifice your own needs for those of others?
7. Who takes care of you? Do they do it well?
8. How do you feel when you think others don't like you or are disappointed with you?
9. What is your greatest fear?
10. What things make you feel guilty?

THE SPECIAL PLACE OF ANGER IN YOUR MEMOIR

Because of its overriding importance, let me repeat a point that I've made several times before in this book: *Anger seems to be the number one emotional culprit in causing the pain and symptoms of AOS.* Anger causes a huge autonomic response; it turns up your inner speedometer quickly and for a long time. Because of this, I want to end with some thoughts that may help you to explore your own anger in your pain memoir.

First, as I've already mentioned in another context, many of my patients have a hard time attaching the word *anger* to themselves. Maybe the emotion just seems too dangerous or socially unacceptable. The term *rage* can carry even more loaded connotations. For example, we may think of violent road-rage incidents where out-of-control drivers start punching or shooting each other.

Many people get a memory block when you tell them to start writing about the anger or rage in their lives. But there is often an easy way out of this impasse. Almost everyone, for instance, will admit to being frustrated or irritated. Exploring those emotions first are often a good way to edge into anger, because they are simply milder forms of anger. In short, if you can't get to first base with your repressed emotions by focusing on anger, try exploring irritation, annoyance, frustration, or disappointment. If you begin your quest this way, you should quickly work your way up to anger, and may even be willing to take a look at the rage in yourself someday.

Here are some depth-journal examples and a daily schedule you might want to use as you move into anger in your journal:

DAYS 1–2 **THE PAST**   EMOTION: **ANGER**

1. What in my past makes me the most angry when I think about it?
2. What about my dad made me angry? What things did he say? What things did he do?
3. Did my parents enjoy me? How did that feel?
4. Was there any abuse—physical, sexual, emotional?
5. What pressure did I feel as a kid?
6. Did I feel unconditionally loved? If not, how did that feel?

DAYS 3–5 PRESENT CIRCUMSTANCES   EMOTION: ANGER

1. What in my current world makes me irritated, frustrated, or angry?
2. What does anger look like in me: hot or cold?
3. What are the three biggest stresses in my life? Write about them.
4. What things can really set me off if I let them?
5. What pressures make me angry?
6. What responsibilities make me angry?
7. How can the ones who love me make me the most angry?

DAYS 6–7 MY PERSONALITY   EMOTION: ANGER

1. What's my pain personality? Am I a Perfectionist? A People-Pleaser? A Legalist? A Stoic? A Fear-Prone personality? A Combo?
2. How does just being me generate a lot of anger during my day?
3. Because of my pain personality, what special pressures do I feel—and how do they make me angry?
4. Because of my pain personality, what do I fear the most—and how does that relate to my anger?

This little exercise will give you a good start delving into repressed anger in your first week of journaling. Next week, you can turn to another dangerous emotion that you suspect might be hiding in your emotional basement. For example, you might focus on fear or shame or one of the many variations on these that we discussed in chapter 4.

Above all, don't get discouraged as you think and write. When you feel you have run out of things to say, start all over on the next page. It's common for patients just beginning a journal to think they have exhausted their storehouse of thoughts and memories after a couple of pages, or even a couple of paragraphs. But then they try again—and again—and inevitably they discover five pages' worth of emotions, or ten, or more. That was my experience, and it well may be yours.

As you uncover these destructive feelings and emotions through the power of depth journaling, you will probably find that you can combine your journal writing quite effectively with another mind–body–spirit method that we introduced in chapter 8—the often dramatic technique that I call pain talk.

10

PAIN TALK

Everything about the man sitting in front of me shouted, *emotional blindness*. He wouldn't acknowledge having anger—or any dangerous emotion, for that matter. I couldn't get him to discuss his emotions at all.

He had flown into Orlando for a consultation about a serious case of chronic back pain, which conventional medicine had been unable to relieve. But as he evaded all my questions about his feelings, and talked only vaguely about his personal background, his family, and his friends, I began to worry about whether I had any chance of helping him. *How am I going to get this guy to understand AOS?* I wondered.

I also suspected that he might have a great deal of trouble developing the important skill that I call pain talk. Over the years, I have become convinced that for the best chance of recovery, *all* of the program steps need to be followed—including pain talk, which is the highlight of Step 2.

Even though I couldn't get this man to open up, I forged ahead, hoping that in some way I might help him find a way to understand AOS. In particular, I wanted him to begin to see his symptoms in terms of their psychological or emotional causes, rather than any physical or structural cause.

From his history with several other physicians, I knew that a wide variety of pain medications had failed to help him. Also, I agreed with his other physicians' conclusions that he was not a candidate for back surgery.

At first, I questioned him about any possible anger or irritation he might be harboring. I knew from my clinical experience that those emotions were most likely to be at the root of his problem. But all I got was a few nods and dismissive gestures.

Then I asked him whether there were any deeply felt spiritual resources that could help him with his symptoms. Again, all I received was shrugs and blank stares. This was not a particularly philosophical or religious guy.

Finally, I talked to him about some of the pain-prone personalities. As close as I could figure, he seemed to fit best into the Stoic personality profile. But he was so reticent to share anything about his life, I couldn't be sure.

This guy is going to have a hard time getting better, I thought. *But I'm sure his symptoms are from Autonomic Overload Syndrome. So I'll have him attend the lecture and maybe he'll pick up something.*

Other patients who were in attendance took seats for the lecture. But this man wanted to stand up in the back corner of the classroom. I think his back may have hurt too much for him to sit down.

During my first lecture, "Anatomy and Physiology of AOS," he paced back and forth across the rear of the lecture room and remained silent. No questions, no comments, no gestures.

Then came the second lecture, where I explain the Pain-Free for Life Treatment Program. I was getting to the part where I said: "You need to take your mind's eye off the physical symptoms and focus it on the subconscious mind, which is keeping you focused on the pain rather than the real culprit, those dangerous emotions. The pain is produced by the subconscious mind in response to a mountain of repressed dangerous emotions for the purpose of keeping your mind's eye *out* of the basement . . ."

Then, almost by accident, I looked directly toward the corner and said toward him, "Anger is most likely at the root of your back pain. The problem is, your subconscious mind is *tricking* you by shifting your anger to the pain in your back—and you don't see it."

He looked at me quietly for a moment and then became visibly irritated.

Uh-oh, I thought. *I've offended him.*

After the lecture was over, he pulled me aside and said: "Hey, Doc, let me get this straight. You telling me my subconscious is trying to con me?"

"Well, that's just my way of—"

"Hold on! You mean I'm really *normal*! No way this [blankety-blank] subconscious is gonna do that! I'll kill it! Absolutely no way any subconscious is gonna fool me into having pain! To [blankety-blank] with that!"

Then I had an idea: "Tell me, how does your back feel—right now?"

He stopped, cocking his head. "I think it feels a lot better, Doc."

I had just witnessed one of the most dramatic and powerful examples of how a person can affect his subconscious mind by talking directly to himself—kicking the pain right out of his back.

All that remained was for me to explain to him in simple terms what he had just accomplished—and how he could continue to use this pain-commanding technique in the future.

Two weeks later I gave him a follow-up call. "Hello, Doc . . . oh yeah, it went away like you said."

"You mean, *totally*?" I said. "When?"

"That day," he said, "I told it to [blankety-blank] and it stopped—it had to. After I realized I was being tricked, I got so mad I cussed at it all the way home. By the time I got home, it was all better. The next day I played tennis, and it hasn't hurt since."

I gave him a follow-up call six weeks later. He was still playing tennis every day and said that if ever his back pain began to resurface, he blasted it verbally, and it promptly disappeared!

Normally, my patients must move carefully through the series of steps outlined in this book over days, weeks, or even a couple of months before they reach the point at which their pain is gone. But this man—through a unique capacity to manhandle his subconscious mind—had short-circuited the overactive autonomic nervous system and achieved instantaneous recovery.

I can't promise such fast relief for you as you develop your pain talk. This patient's case certainly isn't typical. But I can say that learning this mind–body technique will be an invaluable tool in your efforts to banish chronic AOS pain from your life.

PAIN TALK: THE BASICS

Everything in your mind and body talks or communicates. The communication may not be verbal most of the time, but it is communication nevertheless. Millions of small conversations are going on inside your body every minute—shooting back and forth among your inner ear and your cerebellum and your leg muscles so that you remain balanced and don't fall on your face . . . among your brain and eye and tear ducts to make sure your cornea is always clean and moist. As you yell and raise your arm at the guy who just pulled in front of you and cut you off on the highway, messages fly back and forth in your right brain and left brain, your mouth muscles and arm muscles, your heart and pituitary and adrenal glands. Every minute, your mind, body, and spirit are communicating through an "information highway" deep inside.

Pain talk is a mind–body technique that takes advantage of your remarkable inner information highway by establishing a link between your conscious and subconscious minds—and between your conscious thoughts and your autonomic nervous system. Through that communication pathway, you can influence your AOS symptoms with your conscious thoughts, whether spoken or unspoken.

To help you better understand pain talk, here are a few basic principles that have guided my patients during Step 2 of the Pain-Free Program.

PRINCIPLE 1: YOUR CONSCIOUS MIND IS STRONGER THAN YOUR SUBCONSCIOUS MIND

The main treatment principle of mind–body medicine is that your thoughts can exert an influence over your physical body. In AOS, the dangerous emotions in your subconscious mind have overloaded your autonomic nervous system and caused physical symptoms. As a result, you experience pain and other symptoms whenever the autonomic system produces them. In effect, you are out of control, becoming a mere responder to the pain, not a controller of it.

Pain talk helps change all that. Instead of just responding to your pain by running for the heating pad, shifting the back pillow in your seat, or grabbing the pain pills, you use your conscious thoughts to exert an influence over the pain. Over time, and with repetition, you'll learn as I did that you don't have to be passive at all. Your conscious mind can become stronger than the pain-producing subconscious mind. Conscious pain-talk thoughts will override the pain-producing process, and the powerful effect will surprise you—as it once surprised me.

I'll never forget an evening long ago during the six weeks I was battling my own AOS symptoms. My back pain had become about 50 percent better, but that night I began having those dreaded stomach cramps. At first, I wondered if I'd eaten some bad food for lunch, but I quickly recognized my condition as a bout of irritable bowel syndrome (IBS). So off I went to the restroom.

But instead of being a victim of pain for two hours, I began to talk to my subconscious mind, silently but forcefully: "Stop it; stop the squeezing *now*. Relax those bowel muscles. *Relax—stop squeezing now!* I know you're trying to keep me from some dangerous hidden emotion—so I'm going to think about what you're hiding. Stop the pain!"

I thought for a while about what pressure and anger I was feeling. Then I started talking again: "Turn down the speedometer and the cramping *now* . . . you can't distract me with this pain."

Then, after about five minutes, for the first time in my life the cramps began to get less and less severe—and it was over! I came out and shouted to my wife, "Honey, I did it, I made one of the IBS episodes go away—this is unbelievable."

With the Pain-Free Program and the principle of pain talk, Autonomic Overload Syndrome can indeed help patients learn how to make their pain go away—and stay away.

PRINCIPLE 2: PAIN TALK IS CONFRONTATIONAL

As you've probably gathered by now, when you're talking to your subconscious, you must always be firm. The objective is to take control over the subconscious mind's pain production. Your thoughts and pain-talk words should be direct and confident.

I recently asked one of my patients who suffered for years with AOS fibromyalgia symptoms to explain her pain-talk routine. She responded this way: "Anytime I felt a symptom, I would concentrate in my mind on the fact that it was psychological, not physical, and then, you know, I'd rebuke it with my thoughts. I would tell myself that there's really nothing wrong with me, this pain is not a sign of something mysteriously abnormal. Instead, this symptom is like a flashing light on my car dashboard, alerting me to the dangerous emotions lying underneath."

"So would you say that to yourself, or out loud?" I asked.

"Well, both, depending on where I was, and sometimes I would swear at it," she said with a laugh.

With her direct and confident approach, this patient gets her thoughts moving downward into her subconscious mind. While this may sound and feel unusual at first, what is really happening is that, over time, your conscious input into your mind and body are helping you develop stronger, better-conditioned pathways between your conscious thoughts and your subconscious mind. In this way, when you make your demand, the pain process stops.

Another one of my patients describes her pain in these terms: "Every time I get a twinge now, I say to myself, 'Are you kidding me? Do you think I'm an idiot? You can't fool me now. I know what you're trying to hide, and I'm coming down to find out—so stop the pain *now*!'"

Next, this patient enters her subconscious basement, searches for and seizes the hidden negative emotions, and brings them to the conscious level in her mind or in her depth journal. Then she starts asking other pointed questions: *What am I angry about? What pressures do I feel? What responsibility do I feel?*

But a very important question may still be bothering you: *Who am I talking to in pain talk?*

Answer: *To yourself, to your subconscious mind, to your painful areas.*

In other words, this confrontational approach to pain talk can be expressed in almost any way that seems comfortable to you. You can address one, two, or all three of the players in your pain scenario. You can address your pain talk to yourself in general (silently or out loud), or you can address your subconscious mind and demand that it stop the pain or turn down the speedometer. You can also talk directly to the painful areas of your body—a particularly powerful tool when you combine it with your imagination.

PRINCIPLE 3: PAIN TALK INVOLVES
YOUR IMAGINATION

You'll recall that a useful tool for many AOS patients is their imagination. The imagination, like dreams, is a powerful communication pathway in your mind. In fact, dreaming and imagination are similar. In both cases, the mental images that appear frequently result in changes to your autonomic nervous system—so that you may wake up with your heart racing, sweat on your forehead, and real feelings of fear. Or you may have similar responses when your imagination runs wild.

But while you can't control your dreams, you *can* control your imagination, and when you do, the effect on your body can be powerful—and extremely useful in dealing with AOS pain. You can create an image in your mind that relaxes your body, slows your heart rate, and changes your breathing pattern. You can also use your imagination in combination with pain talk to communicate directly with the subconscious mind and painful areas to turn off the pain—as one of my patients does when she experiences any back pain.

"When I use pain talk," she says, "I tell my subconscious mind to turn down the speedometer and stop the pain. I'll also tell the muscles to relax, the blood flow to increase, and the oxygen-rich blood to bathe my muscles and help release the wads of tight muscle fibers. Then I use my imagination to see the muscles starting to relax, and I'll see the speedometer turn down and down until it reaches the relaxed range, or about thirty miles per hour."

In other words, it may help you to create a mental picture while you're using pain talk. In addition to demanding that the subconscious mind stop the pain, you can picture that basement containing your buried emotions, and in your mind's eye *see* yourself rummaging through those old boxes that are crammed with your stuffed feelings.

You're saying to your subconscious (while imagining the picture in your mind), "I'm shutting the door to this deception you're using, where you try to make me believe that there are physical problems with my back. And I'm opening the door to the psychological explanation. I'm going down there to find out what's going on."

PRINCIPLE 4: PAIN TALK AND IMAGINATION COMBINE NATURALLY WITH DEPTH JOURNALING

Pain talk can be used quite effectively both with the imagination *and* with the written word—through your depth journal. To illustrate, suppose you are a Perfectionist personality, and you're writing about the pressure you feel at your job. While you're journaling, you can close your eyes and imagine a day at work:

Visualize your e-mail basket filling up . . . your list of to-dos going on to the sixth page . . . your co-workers taking smoking breaks and not getting any work done . . . your sales for the month being well below forecast . . . and the phone ringing and ringing and ringing. In your mind, see the muscles of your back tightening up and the speedometer in your head turning up to a hundred miles an hour.

Now open your eyes and begin writing what you feel. But instead of just writing about the emotions, write out your pain talk. In your journal, you might jot this down: "Subconscious mind, stop *now*. I'm in control. Stop the pain. I know what you're doing. Muscles, relax *now*. Blood vessels—bring refreshing oxygen to my muscles *now*. Stop the pain *now*."

As you combine these mind–body techniques (visualization, depth journaling, and pain talk), you'll likely notice significant effects and improvements in your body, your mind, and your symptoms.

PRINCIPLE 5: PAIN TALK CONFORMS TO OTHER PROVEN MIND–BODY PREPARATION TECHNIQUES

Some athletes may use related techniques to help them tense up before a contest. You often can see football or basketball players or other team athletes pounding one another's fists, bumping chests, and saying, "Let's go, let's go, let's go!" before they begin a game.

These athletes have learned that through this pumping-up preparation, they can rev up their autonomic nervous systems in ways that are likely to enhance their competitive edge. Among other things, their adrenal glands start pumping out all kinds of epinephrine and other high-performance secretions so that their muscles and brains are ready for action.

Those who want to calm down—such as actors or public speakers before a performance—may reduce their feelings of stress and anxiety by talking to themselves in a soothing verbal rhythm. Each time they breathe out, they may say silently or quietly to themselves, "Calm down, calm down, calm down." Or they may simply concentrate on breathing regularly. Golfers may go through a similar routine just before a high-pressure putt. Through such stress-reduction self-talk techniques, they influence their autonomic nervous systems to lower blood pressure and heart rate, and to release neurotransmitters of well-being, such as endorphins and dopamine.

Pain talk is a mind–body technique that takes the experience of Olympic athletes, sports psychologists, marathon runners, and professional golfers and uses some of their mental strengthening and conditioning insights to reverse the pain-producing process causing AOS symptoms.

PRINCIPLE 6: PAIN TALK IS A CRITICAL PART OF YOUR TREATMENT

Never allow yourself to minimize the use of pain talk or assume that it's some unorthodox practice I invented in my offices at Florida Hospital. Instead, it's a widely used and potent tool in your overall strategy of AOS pain recovery.

In fact, if you do find yourself doubting the power of pain talk, have a heart-to-heart with your subconscious. This sort of uncertainty is just the kind of lie and distraction that the subconscious may use to get your mind off your repressed emotions, which are the real source of your pain.

By verbalizing what you feel, what you want, and what you perceive going on inside your mind and body, you will be in a much stronger position to influence your subconscious mind and, consequently, your mind and body physiology. Or to put this another way, those who talk the pain talk are more likely to enjoy the pain-free walk.

With these basic principles in mind, you're ready to start building your pain vocabulary and fluency with the following pain phrase list.

A SAMPLE PAIN PHRASE LIST

As you begin to develop your own pain-talk tools, here are some suggestions that you might want to use. Or this sample Pain Phrase List may simply stimulate your thinking to help you come up with other words or phrases that work better for you.

- Subconscious, *stop*, you're not tricking me anymore!
- Subconscious, you have no power over my conscious mind.
- Subconscious, from now on I will control you through my conscious thoughts.
- Subconscious, what are you up to?
- Subconscious, what dangerous emotions have you buried?
- Subconscious, turn down my autonomic nervous system *now.*
- Subconscious, I know you're hiding something—you can't fool me.
- Stop the pain in my back *now* (or name whatever AOS pain you have).
- Subconscious mind, I want to dream tonight about the emotions you're so afraid to let out. (This one is powerful at bedtime!)

- I don't have back pain, I have emotional pain. Stop trying to distract me—I know what you're doing.
- There's nothing structurally abnormal with me—I'm normal. I'm healthy, now stop the pain.
- I'm shutting the door to the physical explanations and I'm locking it—I'm coming down into the basement—I'll find out what you're hiding.
- Turn down the autonomic speedometer *now.*
- Bowels, stop squeezing—I know the pain is masking the pressure and anger I'm feeling—so stop *now.* Relax. Relax.
- Blood vessels, relax and dilate and flood the muscles with healing and relaxing blood.

As you grow more fluent in using this pain language, you'll find that the entire treatment plan coalesces into one powerful package. The more you verbalize what you've learned about your pain and yourself, the more you'll continue to learn—and the more likely it will be that you'll find yourself pain-free for life.

THE SEVEN CRUTCHES OF PAIN-PRONE PEOPLE

Now you know how the 6-week Pain-Free for Life Program works, and I'm sure you're eager to get started. But there's another important thing you need to know before you can consider yourself fully equipped to launch into the Pain-Free Program—and that's how to deal with the problem of pain crutches.

Pain crutches are things that you think or things that you do (without even knowing it) that perpetuate the activity of the subconscious mind and keep you from getting better. Or to put it in terms of AOS and the subconscious, *pain crutches are things your subconscious mind relies on in order to keep your pain going.*

Knowing about pain crutches—and how to avoid them—will help prevent any holdups in your recovery from AOS. In this chapter, I'll introduce you to various pain crutches my patients have used *that actually keep them in pain*—and also the techniques you can use to toss them out of your life.

You've no doubt seen people on crutches, and maybe you've had to use them yourself. A crutch is anything you lean or rely on for support. Crutches are certainly useful when you need them to support a healing broken leg. But they are bad if they support and prolong your recovery from chronic pain.

Full recovery from AOS pain is much easier when you recognize what crutches are *holding up your pain*. On the other hand, if you don't see a particular crutch in your life, you probably won't recover as quickly or as fully as you might. And the Autonomic Overload Syndrome will be more likely to give you trouble. In fact, *every one of my AOS patients* has had to deal with one or more pain crutches along the path to recovery.

Sometimes patients whom I've evaluated and diagnosed with Autonomic Overload Syndrome will call to talk about how grateful they are to be "almost" fully recovered from their pain. I'll spend a few minutes asking them questions about their remaining symptoms and their treatment plan. And more often than not, I'll discover that their pain is supported by a pain crutch. Once they realize it, they are free to move forward to complete freedom from pain.

You'll overcome your own crutches with a combination of three things: insight into the identity of your particular pain crutch; an understanding that the crutch won't work; and the courage to throw it away for good.

THE 7 CRUTCHES OF PAIN-PRONE PEOPLE

Here's a list of the top seven pain crutches I see my patients using— or their subconscious minds employing to protect those repressed emotions:

> Crutch 1: The body-medicine crutch.
> Crutch 2: The lack-of-confidence crutch.
> Crutch 3: The medication crutch.
> Crutch 4: The fear crutch.

Crutch 5: The mental diversions crutch.
Crutch 6: The emotional blindness crutch.
Crutch 7: The untreated depression crutch.

These pain crutches *all* have the same effect—perpetuating the ability of the subconscious mind to hide the hidden dangerous emotions by masking them with pain and physical symptoms. Pain crutches keep you from completely closing the door to the physical explanations of your pain: They operate as a kind of wedge stuck under a door that prevents it from closing. To the extent that the door remains open, your AOS symptoms will continue. Let's dispose of each of these crutches in order.

CRUTCH 1: THE BODY-MEDICINE CRUTCH

Mike was a new friend who told me about some lower back pain he had been experiencing for about six months. He had undergone an MRI, which showed a mild to moderate herniated disk in the L4 to L5 area (the area between his fourth and fifth lumbar vertebrae). Mike's orthopedic surgeon assured him that the rest of the MRI of his back looked fine except for this area—so he was a good candidate for surgery. As a result, within a few days of his orthopedic consultation, Mike went under the knife. After surgery, the surgeon confidently announced, "I got it. You shouldn't have any more problems."

It took Mike several months to recover, and during that year, I treated Mike's wife for the AOS symptom of fibromyalgia. Kathy was a wonderful patient and a firm believer in her AOS diagnosis and treatment plan. In fact, she completely recovered from all her symptoms in about six weeks. During her recovery, Mike talked about how incredibly Kathy was doing, and how it had changed her (and their) life.

"I hate to say the program worked like magic," her husband said. "But in many ways, it really did. Only about five days after Kathy heard your first lecture, she was symptom-free. It was unbelievable. The cure didn't take months or years. It was less than a week."

But when it came to his own back, well, that was another story. "Oh, that was different," he said. "I had a herniated disk, not Autonomic Overload Syndrome. Besides, I'm out of pain."

Although he gave lip service to his support of Kathy's diagnosis and treatment plan, Mike didn't believe this "emotions stuff" could possibly apply to him. Kathy and I would sometimes joke about Mike—calling him an "AOS dabbler." He toyed with the idea, but when it came to himself, it didn't seem to apply.

About a year later, Mike began to get some back pain again, but another MRI revealed no new herniations. One afternoon, when I dropped by his office to take him to lunch, I noticed he was hobbling around, gently moving and picking things up with one hand and tightly holding his lower back. When I asked him about his pain, he knew where I was going.

"I know, but it's not *that*," he said, waving me off. "I hurt it windsurfing with my daughter. It'll go away."

Hundreds of pills, several doctor visits, and hours of heating pads later, he found he felt better. Still, for the next couple of years, he went in and out of back pain episodes, which typically lasted two to three weeks then let up.

The following summer, Mike called me while he was on vacation: "Hey, Doc, I'm really hurting. One of my back episodes is ruining my vacation. Do you *really* think it's AOS?"

"I've known you for a while now," I replied. "You're a Perfectionist, you're a Stoic, and you're a professional emotion repressor. Your MRI didn't show anything new. So yes, I do think you have AOS."

Reluctantly, he decided to ask his wife to lead him through the Pain-Free for Life Treatment Program, which she knew by heart.

When he got back from vacation, he proudly announced, "You won't believe it, or, actually you *will* believe it. I'm all better, I made it go away. The pain is completely gone! I was able to do anything I wanted on vacation—including mountain hiking, water-skiing, and windsurfing. Now, you can't do that with a *weak back*, can you! Sometimes I'd get a little twinge, but I would do the treatment in my mind and within a couple of minutes I could make the pain disappear. Doc, you were right—this stuff is powerful medicine."

For several years—despite seeing the power of the Pain-Free Program right before his eyes, as his wife recovered from years of chronic fibromyalgia pain—he couldn't get over his body-medicine crutch. He couldn't believe anything except the propaganda tapes that were playing so loudly in the living room of his mind: *You've got a bad back, it's a disk, don't lift too much, you're abnormal.*

Now, I'm not saying that Mike's first surgery was definitely unnecessary. He may have had a severe disk extrusion or a bony fragment. But his body-medicine crutch got worse after the surgery because he had begun to believe firmly that his back was weak and prone to injury. This mind-set provides a perfect thought pattern to give the subconscious mind a means to send more pain symptoms and hide dangerous emotions.

With the body-medicine crutch, Mike's subconscious mind was able to cover up the threatening emotions that had built up over time. His mountain of repressed emotions had overloaded his autonomic nervous system to the point that he had begun to develop muscle tightness and lower back pain. But all he could think about was his structurally "weak" back. The pain, along with the body-medicine crutch, kept him completely unaware of the dangerous emotions.

In effect, his mind's eye *never* looked down into the subconscious mind, because his crutch conditioned him to *know* that he had something physically or structurally wrong with him. Largely because of that crutch—and his body-medicine belief that backs are weak and all back pain is structural in nature—it took him years to get to his aha moment with AOS.

Like Mike, most AOS patients come to see me after they've had pain for years and after they've generally had many physician consultations. Their mind is filled with body-medicine conclusions given to them by well-meaning but narrowly focused medical professionals.

If you're using this body-medicine crutch, by the way, you should know that it's very common to hear the body-medicine tapes in your mind quite loudly when you begin trying the AOS Pain-Free for Life Program. In order to get better, AOS patients with this crutch must concentrate diligently on Step 1 of the program—closing the door to the physical explanations of their pain.

Of course, you must always see your local physician when you have any physical symptoms—including pain. But keep an open mind, and ask your physician questions about whether or not you have any definitive structural abnormality. In other words, don't conclude automatically that your body is weak and abnormal.

CRUTCH 2: THE LACK-OF-CONFIDENCE CRUTCH

The second most common crutch I see among AOS recovering patients—one that the subconscious mind can use quite effectively—is a struggle with confidence. Some have a difficult time building confidence in their diagnosis of AOS because their local physician has never mentioned it, and it goes against the conventional medical grain.

Many AOS sufferers will read this book, experience the aha moment of insight, apply the Pain-Free for Life Program, and get better in forty days. But others need to have me or another mind–body–spirit physician look them directly in the eye and say, "Yes, you've got AOS." That's the only way they will develop enough confidence to get better. You can also boost your confidence by seeing your own local physician and being reassured that he or she can find *no* correctable structural abnormalities with your body.

This crutch may emerge in fence-straddling patients who say, "I'll give this Pain-Free Program a try for a few days or maybe a week, but I really have my doubts about it."

Or others might express their reservations this way: "I'm a practical-minded, scientifically oriented kind of person. I really don't think I have the kind of personality that will fit this program. But I'll look it over for a few days . . ."

Still others will read this book and have an aha moment as they identify with almost everything in this book. That initial response will help them take giant steps toward pain relief. But when they tell a friend, neighbor, or local physician about the program—and they get a skeptical reaction—it breaks their confidence like a piece of fine china, and their pain goes downhill from there. That was the case with a patient of mine named Carol.

CAROL'S CRUTCHES

Carol, an extremely busy mother of three small children, began to experience a nagging pain in one knee when she was in her late thirties. As a result, she couldn't maneuver around the house as easily as before.

"When I'd go upstairs, it really hurt," she recalled. "At first, one knee seemed to be hurting more than the other. So I would walk just one step at a time, carefully lifting the bad leg up and putting it down. That really bothered me because I'm not that old. I thought, *This is not good.*"

As she tried to be more careful in her movements, things steadily got worse rather than better. "I started to have problems just moving around on flat surfaces around the house. So I'd try to kind of take things easier. I wouldn't be as active with my kids and my family."

One day, while she was playing at a party with her children, she felt shooting pains in her knees and shoulders. "They didn't last long, but they were sharp enough to make me realize that something wasn't right."

Soon Carol decided that she would have to give up her regular walking routine because she feared that the exercise might hurt her body even more. "Being a mom of young kids, I can't afford to not feel good," she said. "If I can't move about, I can't be a good mother."

Then she began to have a recurrence of jaw pains that had bothered her when she was wearing braces in college. So she went to her dentist, who fitted her for a bite plate—and mentioned the words *TMJ syndrome*. His analysis was that her jaw pain had to be the result of her grinding her teeth while she was asleep. The bite plate, he said, would help provide some relief during the night.

Then her other aches and pains seem to grow worse: "One morning I woke up and had a zinging pain, a shooting pain going down the back of my leg, a nerve pain. I thought, *What was that?* At first, I ignored it, but later in the day, I had another. That started happening over and over, many times a day."

Soon she began to worry that she had some sort of serious disease or that "something is really wrong with me."

Carol was the type of person who knew everyone in her town, including several physicians. Her friends gave her lots of different homespun diagnoses, and her physicians concluded that she had fibromyalgia, gastritis, irritable bowel syndrome, sciatic neuralgia, migraine headaches, and TMJ syndrome. She had tried "everything," including years of failed medications, exercises, weight loss, heating pads, and the bite plate. Then she got my name from a friend of a friend whom I had helped cure.

After giving her a thorough medical exam, I looked at her X-rays and took an extensive psychological, physical, and spiritual history.

During our interview, it was very easy to see that Carol was a People-Pleaser personality who had a profound need to keep everyone in her orbit of family and friends happy. With lots of kids and tons of friends, she could never live up to the standards she felt others wanted of her. As a result, she was constantly under stress and regularly stuffed unpleasant emotions, such as anxiety, disappointment (that is, anger), irritation (that is, anger), guilt, and fear.

Carol was a wonderful patient. She quickly grasped the concept of AOS and the Pain-Free Treatment Program. Also, she immediately agreed with my assessment that there were no physical structural abnormalities that would explain her pain. She accepted that her pain was rooted in buried emotions and that a mind–body–spirit approach could cure her completely.

After she had been on the program for a couple of weeks, she reported significant progress: "The other day, I thought, *I haven't had one of those zinging pains in my knees or down my leg in the last six hours.* That was exciting!"

Over the next week or so, as a "sort of gradual thing," she said, "my knees slowly improved, and the pain just started to go away."

After about a month, she said, "I've been feeling very good. I haven't had any more knee pain at all. Those zinging pains have disappeared. Once in a while, at the very beginning, I would have a mild recurrence. But eventually, there was absolutely no pain at all."

Carol was well on her way to enjoying life again. But then she began sharing her story with her friends. She listened to every friend's disbelief and skepticism with open ears—mostly, I think, because of her desire to make her friends happy. One friend mentioned that she knew someone with a condition just like Carol's—and it turned out to be cancer! Another said that despite feeling better, she shouldn't overdo it.

Soon afterward, Carol got another mild AOS pain. She saw her local physician, who ended up scolding her for not wearing her knee brace and for taking out her bite plate. Her confidence was shot! For the next six months, Carol spiraled down back into chronic multiple pains.

When I finally spoke with her, I was amazed at how quickly she had lost confidence in her AOS diagnosis and gone back to the old explanations for her pain. She had even restarted all the old treatments that never worked in the first place.

The last time I spoke with Carol, she was back on track and 85 percent of her symptoms were gone. But much to my disappointment, I could still detect in her voice the lack-of-confidence crutch that will most likely continue to haunt her and keep her from becoming completely pain-free.

CRUTCH 3: THE MEDICATION CRUTCH

Assume that you've decided you might have AOS, you've discussed it with your doctor, and you've begun the 6-week Pain-Free for Life Program. In that case, I would like you to remain on the same pain-associated medications you have been taking for at least three to four weeks.

This waiting period will give you time to focus on the program without having to mix in the issues related to weaning and stopping medicines. Also, I've instructed you to change your medications *only* under the guidance of your local physician and to continue taking those medications you're using for medical problems such as diabetes, high blood pressure, cancer, high cholesterol, or arthritis. This particular crutch does *not* refer to these types of medicines (I'm only talking about pain medications here).

Medications can be wonderful things when you have pain. However, it's easy to begin to rely on this crutch as a necessary supplement to the Pain-Free for Life Program, and once that happens, the power of the program diminishes significantly.

After diagnosing one patient with Autonomic Overload Syndrome, I asked him about his medications. His chart listed Tylenol as the only medication he took.

Then he said, "I'm on vitamins, too. Is it okay for me to keep taking my vitamins?"

I asked, "Why are you taking them?"

He thought for a moment and replied, "I think they're good for my health. And they make me feel better and give me more energy, especially the vitamin C."

"Okay, now be completely honest with me," I said. "Are you taking the vitamins, at least in part, because you think the vitamins may help your back or your headaches?"

Note: The answer to this particular question determines whether the vitamin is a crutch or not. Specifically, a *yes* or *maybe* means you're dealing with a crutch. A definite *no* means it's probably not a crutch.

His answer? After a couple of seconds and then a sheepish grin, he responded, "Maybe."

"Then you're dealing with a crutch," I said. "You've got to stop the vitamins for forty days. After that, assuming you are convinced in your own mind that vitamins have nothing to do with your pain relief, you can start back on them."

Although I'm a believer in one-a-day multivitamins, his vitamins were keeping the door to the physical answers to his pain (his "living room") open. He was taking the vitamins to help the pain, but they were actually *preventing* him from getting better on the Pain-Free for Life Program as quickly as he should because they prevented him from focusing his mind's eye *exclusively* on the repressed subconscious emotions.

During my own recovery, the medication crutch held me up for a few weeks. I had stopped my pain medications, but I still kept the pills in my vanity drawer. I'd been off them for a week or two, but subconsciously I couldn't get up the courage to throw them all away, "just in case this program doesn't do the job completely."

Finally I opened the vanity drawer while looking for my razor one day, and it occurred to me, *Now's the time Scott—it's either physical or psychological—you're either in or out.* I knew I was *in.* So I threw away the medicines—every one of them. And guess what happened? My pain increased for the next three days! It must have been the last stand for my subconscious mind, one last effort to wreck my confidence and get my focus out of the subconscious basement and back to the physical symptoms.

But after those three days, I began a fairly rapid recovery and soon reached the point where I've remained for years—pain-free.

EXERCISE AS A MEDICATION CRUTCH

Exercise can work as a pain crutch in much the same way as pills. I always ask my physically active or athletic AOS patients, "Why are you exercising?"

If the answer is, "Because it makes my back feel better," or something close to that, I have a standard—and, I must admit, a rather radical-sounding—response:

"If you are exercising because you think that it's going to cause your back to get any better, then you have to *stop* exercising until you understand that it's absolutely necessary to *shut the door* on any physical explanations or physical cures for your pain."

Now, I can already hear the objections from other physicians, especially those who are fitness or preventive medicine experts: "But regular exercise is essential for a person's health—to prevent heart disease, reduce the odds of all-cause mortality, and strengthen bones and muscles as we age!"

All that is absolutely true, and I am not, by any means, suggesting that you or any other patient should swear off exercise for the rest of your life. Rather, I direct my patients who rely on exercise to help their pain to stop that activity for the duration of the 6-week program. Then, once the pain has improved without exercise and they finally understand the power of thinking psychologically, it's fine to resume exercise, vitamins, or whatever (but not pain medication!).

Of course, many AOS patients *do not* exercise, take vitamins, or engage in other activities for the purpose of helping their pain. In that case, I tell them just to keep on doing what they're doing. The mind–body–spirit treatment won't be adversely affected in those situations.

CRUTCH 4: THE FEAR CRUTCH

The fear crutch, which is very common among people who've been in pain for a long time, can trip up AOS patients in at least two different ways. One way is that they set out to resume physical activity, then can't find the courage to go through with it, because they fear it might set them back. This is a *specific-fear crutch*.

So a person may avoid tennis or golf, saying, "Tennis will hurt me—especially the serving, or the quick starting and stopping." Or, as I used to say about golf, "The twisting of my back and upper body is sure to make my back pain worse."

Even after a patient begins to understand that repressed dangerous emotions—and not any structural problem—are causing the pain, there may be a reluctance to try the old activity. That's why I always encourage my patients who are experiencing little or no pain after a few weeks of the program to begin resuming *all* normal physical activity—because their physical body really is normal.

I tell them, "Hey, you can go ahead and play golf, or sit any way you like in your car, or plan on watching an entire movie. Your body is normal!"

I go on to explain, "If your subconscious mind tries to deceive you and produce pain, don't be afraid! You can bet you'll be able to resume your regular, favorite sports and other activities if you just recognize those fears have no power over you."

The second type of fear crutch is the *generalized-fear crutch.* This crutch typically involves a general fear that your body is weak and easily injured. I see this in a lot of patients who have suffered the multiple AOS pain symptoms of fibromyalgia, such as a young woman by the name of Kay.

KAY CASTS OFF HER FEAR CRUTCH

Kay, a recent college graduate, had been struggling with debilitating pain for about ten years. Her symptoms involved pain in her feet, neck, and shoulders, and she also suffered from generalized body aches and headaches. The aches exhausted her to the point that a couple of days a week, she felt as though she were coming down with the flu.

"I'd sometimes go to my doctor, but then the symptoms would disappear soon after I returned home," she recalled.

Finally, a physician diagnosed her with fibromyalgia, which is characterized by generalized muscle aches and pains. He prescribed some medicines, but "they made me feel out of it," she said. "So I quit taking them and tried to deal with the pain on my own."

A series of cortisone shots helped her pain temporarily. But when the effects wore off, the pain returned. Everything in her life was now a huge effort as she attempted to fulfill her duties as a youth leader and a college student.

"Some days my schedule seemed so overwhelming that I couldn't even get up," she said. "I just stayed in bed."

To top off her problems, she began to develop irritable bowel syndrome (IBS), including indigestion problems, which constantly disrupted her life. Sometimes she would have to skip classes, and even tests, to go to the bathroom. Things had reached the point that she was reluctant to go out with her friends for fear of having to be in the bathroom for a couple of hours with IBS cramps.

Her doctors predicted that she would have the fibromyalgia

symptoms "for the rest of her life" and that she would just have to try to manage the pain as best she could. "There's no cure," one doctor told her. Steadily, she became convinced that she was weak and physically frail.

"Whenever I stayed out past midnight, I would pay for it the next couple days with worse neck and backaches," she recalled. "I became afraid to *push it* . . . afraid that my body couldn't take it."

She continued to shop around for solutions, including bone-manipulation sessions with chiropractors. But the symptoms remained as bad as ever, and they began to travel to other parts of the body. She would deal with severe migraines for a period of time, and then, just as those seemed to get better, her lower back would hurt more. And before long, there would be another round of IBS symptoms.

"It was like some kind of gopher game," she said. "Just as it seemed I might be getting on top of one thing, another symptom would pop up somewhere else. It seemed like the problems were never going to end."

At that point, Kay decided to look me up.

Kay was a great student of AOS. Within weeks her symptoms began to go away. I remember a phone call a couple of weeks after I saw her: "I did it! I actually aborted a migraine headache!"

She continued to drink in the information, and as she absorbed fact after fact, her belief in the program and its ability to help her grew stronger and stronger. So Kay continued to study, listen to my taped lectures, and assimilate the information that was relevant to her various complaints. Her symptoms continued to resolve, but her progress was slower than I hoped—so we talked.

"Kay, how's the program going?" I asked.

"Great, I'm doing everything we talked about," she replied.

"It's been six weeks now—have you started enjoying life again?" I asked.

As we talked, her fear crutch became clear. "Well, I mainly stay around the dorm room and read and do the program. I'm afraid to really push it; whenever I've tried to keep up with my girlfriends in the past, I've paid for it the next few days—I'm just very afraid."

Kay had done everything just right on the program, but she stumbled for a few weeks over the fear crutch. She had considered her physical body weak for as long as she could remember, and when she got a diagnosis of fibromyalgia, it just reinforced her fear that she was physically abnormal.

But as I said, Kay was a great student. She recognized that her fear was perpetuating her symptoms by keeping her focused on the physical rather than the psychological. Before long, she became downright confident that her physical body was normal and strong—and within several weeks, her symptoms made amazing improvements.

CRUTCH 5: THE MENTAL DIVERSIONS CRUTCH

When you have chronic pain, there are probably many habits and diversions in your lifestyle that can become a crutch—including practices or routines you avoid, or superstitions you honor because somehow you think that they will help your pain. Here are a few of these diversions:

- If I sleep with this pillow between my legs, it helps my back pain.
- If I jog in the morning I'm okay, but if I don't, I'll hurt more.
- If I sleep on my left side, it won't hurt my spine.
- If I wear these shoes rather than those shoes, I am going to be okay.
- If I don't walk on hard surfaces, I won't hurt my back as much.

- If I sleep with a heating pad on my back every night, I'll feel better.
- If I don't wear high heels, I won't hurt.
- If I put a pillow behind my back when I drive, I'm okay.
- If I stretch my legs every morning, my back won't be as bad.
- I'm going to hurt more tonight because I'm not on my good mattress.

Chronic AOS pain can hurt so badly that we're sometimes willing to believe or do almost anything to get rid of it. In effect, we develop habits and superstitions that probably have helped the pain a little in the past. The habits seem innocent—and often make sense. But they only serve to help deceive us into thinking that our bodies are weak, frail, and prone to pain with the least little thing. They divert us from the real cause of pain, which lies in those repressed emotions.

At this point, you may want to jot down all those little habits, superstitions, and other diversions that may be getting in the way of curing your chronic AOS pain. You once thought that you needed them. But now you understand that these crutches only help prolong the pain—so get rid of them!

CRUTCH 6: THE EMOTIONAL BLINDNESS CRUTCH

Although 85 percent of my patients have significant to complete pain improvement in six to eight weeks, the other 15 percent seem to say some very similar things: "I'm no good at journaling—I can't write—it's not my thing." Or, "I've been writing for a couple weeks, and I just can't get anything." Or, "I'm just not an angry kind of person—at least not the way you're describing it."

Behind each of these statements is a common thread: *No way do I have a mountain of dangerous negative emotions like anger (cer-*

*tainly not rage!). That's just not me. I'm not perfect, but I don't
struggle with anger like some folks do.*

Maybe you haven't spoken those exact words, but the thoughts
come across just as clearly.

I see this crutch used a lot among patients who are highly religious. You've probably figured out by now that I have a strong personal faith and spiritual commitment. So I'm speaking here as both
a physician observer of patients who use this crutch—as well as the
strongest of offenders who uses this crutch himself!

Religious people are often the best emotional pretenders. It's
our goal to be nice and sweet and loving and compassionate. So
when we find out that we really aren't as nice as we should be, the
most common path taken is to ignore reality and pretend that we're
different from the person we really are. I sometimes tell patients
like these, "Emotional pretending perpetuates pain!"

As you know, part of my office visit includes taking a spiritual history. When I find people who say that their faith is very important
to them, I'll begin probing to see if they have any clue about the
narcissistic and sinful lower nature—known as the "flesh" in biblical terminology. On occasion, I'll find out that people like this are
fairly insightful about themselves, warts and all. But usually, these
types engage in a lot of self-deception and pretending in order to
keep up the religious facade.

Of course, highly spiritual people aren't the only emotional pretenders in life. Another category of my patients—men in their late
fifties and older—are frequently emotionally blind. For some reason, to talk and think and write about emotions is completely foreign to many of them.

For example, I'll get through the first hour-long lecture on the
anatomy and physiology of Autonomic Overload Syndrome, and
these men will hang in there with me—asking great questions and
nodding frequently. About halfway through the second lecture,
however, when I'm talking about the treatment plan, mind–body

techniques, and depth journaling, it's common to see a glazed look beginning to move across their eyes, or see them start glancing at their wives as if they are signaling: *Emotions? . . . Anger? . . . What's he talking about? . . . That's not me!*

If you're prone to this crutch, and emotions are something you generally avoid, I've found that just *talking* with a spouse or close friend (who is willing to be honest about your warts) is a very helpful plan of attack. The approach often gets the emotional discovery juices flowing. Before you know it, you find you are talking through some very significant repressed dangerous emotions that you've dug up and brought out.

CRUTCH 7: THE UNTREATED DEPRESSION CRUTCH

Jennifer was only twenty-eight, but she had nagging lower back pain going on ten years. Her dad and brother were physicians, and they both agreed that she should come see me for a visit. Her doctor had done extensive medical evaluations including MRIs and blood tests to rule out dangerous conditions, but everything had come out normal. At the time of her visit, she was having pain in her right lower back and pegged it as a seven on a scale of one to ten.

As I always do when I evaluate patients for AOS, I spent about forty-five minutes with Jennifer, asking her lots of questions about her physical symptoms; her personality; and her medical, family, social, psychological, and spiritual history. I also performed a physical exam (she was normal), and then we ventured back to my office to discuss her condition.

Although she seemed to be a classic case of Autonomic Overload Syndrome, her pain clearly wasn't the only thing that was wrong with her. She looked sad, her face was drawn, and she showed very little expression during my history taking. I asked her if she felt depressed, and I could tell that my question had struck a chord.

"I don't know," she replied. "Yes, I've thought about it. But none of my doctors has ever said anything to me about it. I don't always feel sad, but today is a hard day."

I shifted gears from AOS and began probing her with questions related to depression and dysthymia (mood disorder). Finally, I concluded that Jennifer was depressed and needed medication for her depression.

In Jennifer's case, she needed two treatments: medication for her depression and the Pain-Free for Life Program for her AOS lower back pain.

A PRIMER ON DEPRESSION

Depression is actually a group of disorders that includes major depression, dysthymia, and bipolar (manic-depression) disorder. Depression is very common, but it's estimated that 80 percent of people who suffer go undiagnosed and untreated. Here are a few other sobering statistics:

* One in five women will develop clinical depression sometime in her life.
* Sixteen percent of all adults will experience depression.
* Depression affects about fourteen million American adults *every year*.
* Depression can quadruple your risk of dying after a heart attack.

People with depression are at higher risk for almost every medical condition, including heart disease, chronic pain, and suicide. The condition involves more than just feeling down in the dumps for a few days. Rather, there is a feeling of being down, or even hopeless, for weeks at a time. If you have any of the following symptoms of depression, you should see your local physician for an evaluation:

- Depressed or irritable mood almost every day.
- Persistent sad, anxious, or "empty" mood.
- Feelings of worthlessness or helplessness.
- Loss of interest or pleasure in activities that you once enjoyed.
- Inability to sleep or sleeping too much.
- Agitation or restlessness.
- Loss of energy or constant fatigue.
- Difficulty concentrating or making decisions.
- Thoughts of death or suicide.

Warning: If you or someone you know has thoughts of suicide, consider it a medical emergency that must be taken seriously. Please call your doctor *today* or go to the nearest hospital for help.

Dysthymia, one of the conditions Jennifer was examined for in the above example, is a milder type of depression. It's not something that hits all of a sudden, but instead seems to creep up on you. The problem often lasts for several years before it's noticed. Many times, patients I diagnose with dysthymia will say, "I don't feel a lot different than I usually feel. I'm kind of irritable, but that's just me. If I think back a few years, though, I can remember being happier, more carefree, lighter, and less irritable."

Warning signs for dysthymia include:

- Increased irritability (easily angered).
- Conflicts with family and friends.
- Withdrawal from social events and people.

About 3 percent of people will suffer dysthymia at some time in their lives. Like major depression, dysthymia is twice as likely to appear in women as in men. Symptoms usually emerge in young adulthood, but in some cases the symptoms don't show up until middle age.

DEPRESSION AND CHRONIC PAIN

Depression is one of the most common problems experienced by patients with chronic pain. I've noticed that about 20 to 25 percent of my AOS patients have at least mild to moderate depression or dysthymia, and many times the conditions go undiagnosed despite multiple physician visits. (I refer to this link between depression and chronic pain to indicate that there is definitely an *association* between the two. That is, where you find one, you often find the other. Furthermore, in individual patients, AOS may operate to help cause depression.)

Diagnosing depression in people with chronic pain is sometimes difficult because the symptoms can overlap. In an eight-year study, the National Center for Health Statistics found that depressed patients were twice as likely to develop chronic pain as nondepressed individuals.[1] Another study found that in people with unexplained chronic back pain, 66 percent had a history of recurrent depression compared to less than 20 percent of those without pain.[2]

The untreated depression pain crutch is a little different from the rest of the crutches because depression is a chemical disorder rather than a habit, thought, or action. Nevertheless, like all crutches, if depression remains undiagnosed and unaddressed, it will keep you from recovering from AOS as rapidly or as completely as you otherwise could.

These depression-related conditions are frequently associated with large amounts of strong negative emotions, including guilt, anxiety, anger, and irritability. Like the pain-prone personalities that cause lots of strong negative emotions, depression and dysthymia can cause individuals to experience an overload of dangerous emotions. In addition, these conditions make it difficult for your mind to focus and concentrate when you're doing the Pain-Free Program.

. . .

Now, as we draw near the end of this description of the Autonomic Overload Syndrome and the treatment plan I employ to treat it, I'm sure you have some questions. So let's spend a little time together as I field some of the most common queries I hear in my office and at my lectures.

12

DR. BRADY FIELDS
YOUR QUESTIONS

As each patient's treatment program unfolds, questions inevitably come to mind. Here are some that I hear most often—and how I respond.

QUESTION: How long does it take to get better?

ANSWER: It's been my experience that it takes about four to six weeks for most AOS patients to have significant improvement. About three-quarters of our patients will get at least 80 percent better within four to six weeks. Some people get better a lot quicker, and a smaller percentage of people can take eight or ten weeks to get better. The pattern for improvement is different for everyone, but it's common to follow the two-steps-forward-and-one-step-back pattern. When I began the program myself, my symptoms got *worse* for the first few weeks—because I was delving into some strong negative emotions that kicked up a lot of autonomic activation. Don't get discouraged—press on!

QUESTION: What can help AOS patients get better more quickly?

ANSWER: In addition to understanding and following the treatment plan as outlined in this book, there are three things that influence your recovery:

* Confidence in your diagnosis of AOS. A small percentage of AOS patients will not get better quickly because they lack confidence in their diagnosis. When they leave my office, they're confident in their diagnosis, but after they get home they begin to worry about the "crooked back" diagnosis they received from their chiropractor. Or when they talk with a friend, they become sure the pain is from a bone spur.

* Your ability to shut the door completely to the physical explanations and treatments for your chronic AOS pain. When you let the door remain open a bit (such as by using pain crutches, or by lack of confidence in your diagnosis), your subconscious mind will continue to produce the symptoms in an attempt to keep you from delving exclusively into the basement of your emotions.

* Your openness and insightfulness with yourself as you begin to think about those repressed strong negative emotions. Remember, you repressed these emotions on purpose (even though the process may not have been conscious) because they were dangerous and threatening. It's not easy seeing things about yourself that you don't like. Have courage!

QUESTION: When I write my pain journal, should I write down things I remember only one time—but not write them down the next day if I remember them again?

ANSWER: The object is not to find a hundred buried emotions and get them all out on a piece of paper in the form of a hundred short sentences. The object is to remember the emotion and experience it as much as possible as you journal. Do your journaling thoughtfully, slowly, and deeply. If you think about it again tomorrow—write about it some more. Most likely, you'll find something different the next time you write about it.

A special note: If you're dealing with devastating, life-changing memories, such as rape, divorce, or parental suicide, please seek the help of a trained psychologist to process these thoughts if you haven't already done so. Memories and experiences as serious as these are best processed with the help of someone who is trained to do so.

QUESTION: When can I consider myself normal?

ANSWER: I consider my patients normal or recovered when they experience minimal or no pain, when any minor symptoms don't interfere with their life, and when they are able to resume all normal physical activities.

A major ingredient in complete AOS recovery is that you have to overcome your fear, such as fear of playing golf because it twists your back, or fear of overdoing it because "it" might worsen your fibromyalgia. Your subconscious mind uses your fear to keep you away from the dangerous emotions. But fear contributes to your pain and increases it. In other words, if you give in to the fear of making certain movements or exposing yourself to certain situations, the pain will probably return. But when you rob that fear of its power—with such tools as pain talk and journaling—your confidence will grow. And your pain should get better and better.

QUESTION: Do I need to quit my stressful job?

ANSWER: Once patients learn that the stresses and pressures in their lives—including that in their jobs—contribute to a lot of their pain, they wonder if they should quit for a while.

I tell them, "Don't quit your job because of AOS. You're always going to encounter stresses and pressures in your life no matter what job you have."

Remember, its not the job stress that's the problem—it's those dangerous repressed emotions! For that matter, all serious endeavors in life carry the possibility of stress. You can have the best marriage in the world, for instance, but all good and deep relationships will involve stress and difficult times.

Always keep in mind that *the cause of your AOS pain is not the pressure or the stress that always bears down upon you. Rather, the cause is the repressed emotions that have resulted from the way you handle your stress.* So your focus should not be on escaping all stress but on controlling the repressive tendencies and identifying and expressing your emotions appropriately, without burying them. Remember, it's only "professional repressors" who get AOS!

QUESTION: Should I keep seeing my personal physician, who has treated me for these headaches and fibromyalgia for a long time, even though I'm embarking on your program?

ANSWER: The answer is absolutely *yes.* Tell your doctor about your new approach to the symptoms and feel free to give him or her all the materials you've received from us, including this book.

Most doctors intrinsically understand that there are connections among stress, emotions, and physiological changes. But medical school hasn't taught any of us how to effectively diagnose and solve these types of problems. Still, I rarely find doctors who are negative toward patients wishing to pursue mind–body treatments.

I ask my patients to *always* follow up with their primary care physicians—even though their AOS symptoms can be cured with our program, we all get sick or injured in other ways eventually. I don't want anyone to read this book and embark on the program without first making sure that their pain isn't caused by a dangerous or emergency condition! So please be sure to follow up with your regular doctor. Also, if you experience any new pains or if your current pain changes in any way, you should be evaluated further by your local physician.

QUESTION: I once loved to work out every day. When can I start exercising regularly again?

ANSWER: I ask all my AOS patients to wait about three to four weeks before they get involved again in the full routine of jogging, golf, tennis, or whatever it is that they have stopped. It usually takes that long for the pains to begin to subside significantly. If the pains continue to the point that it really hurts to exercise, I may recommend staying even six weeks or longer on the treatment plan before strenuous workouts.

The main reason for delaying a while with the exercise is that I want patients to build up some confidence in the Pain-Free for Life Program before they plunge completely into their rigorous activity. As I said above, it's very common for our subconscious mind to heighten or intensify the pain during those activities. The objective for the subconscious—if I may personify our main pain opponent again—is to try to convince you, *Oh, there it is again! My back was better, but I really* do *have a weak physical body. It's not those emotions after all.*

That's what happened to me with golf. As you know, I discovered that I had AOS-induced chronic back pain. With the treatment plan I was getting better and better, to the point that my pain had mostly disappeared. But as soon as I started playing golf again, my back tightened up like a three-cord rope, and I thought, *Oh no, I've ruined it!* My mind raced with disappointment, my confidence in the AOS diagnosis was shaken, and I was so mad that I had ruined weeks of having only minimal pain.

Then I remembered: *Oh, yeah, that's right! The subconscious mind is still trying to keep me away from these dangerous negative repressed emotions by giving me these physical pains.* I focused on the repressed emotions, hit more golf balls, and the pain went away.

In other words, I was far enough along in my treatment that I had the confidence and skill to shift my mind-set back to a productive mind–body strategy. So I usually ask AOS patients to do the treatment plan for three to four weeks before they venture into the next stage of resuming those activities that they have stopped.

QUESTION: When should I stop my pain medication?

ANSWER: AOS patients should wait awhile before tapering off their pain medications, especially if they are on narcotics. It takes a lot of mental energy and concentration to begin to look down inside yourself at those dangerous emotions and then start pulling them out. Pain takes away your ability to think and concentrate.

To give yourself a clear mental focus and the concentration to complete the program, I say go ahead and stay on your medicines for three to four weeks. After that, *under the direction of your local doctor* (especially if you have been on pain medicines for a long time), you can start weaning yourself from those medicines.

In any event, please do *not* stop pain medications all at once. If you stop your medications cold turkey, you may go through some withdrawal symptoms and additional bouts with physical pain, which will keep you so preoccupied with the pain that it will be hard to make it through the treatment plan.

Caution: Remember that if you are using medicines for reasons other than AOS pain—such as for high blood pressure, high cholesterol, or diabetes—you *must* continue with those medications.

QUESTION: I have told several friends and family members about how I've gotten better from ten years of back pain with your program and about how I think it's a miracle. But I am finding that people are not apt to listen. They tend to be very skeptical. Why is that?

ANSWER: I hear this a lot—and it is frustrating! There are several reasons:

First, we Americans have been brainwashed into believing that our backs are weak and that our back pain is caused by physical lifting, twisting, or pulling. We're told over and over, "Bend your knees when you lift or it will hurt you." So the standard response to hearing about AOS for the first time is usually skepticism.

Second, we like a quick fix, including taking pills as a "cure." Unfortunately, people don't understand that pain pills do not cure: they're just temporary relief methods that don't go to the root of the problem. That's why the problems come back over and over again. After the medication wears off, the symptoms typically return.

Another reason for the skepticism is that emotions are taboo to many people. When you try to explain to people that your problem—or theirs—might lie in the emotions, they start thinking: "Oh no, that might work for you, but I've got *real* pain . . . it started after I lifted . . . you don't understand . . . I don't have any emotional issues . . . I am just not that kind of person."

If you begin to explain the pain problems in terms of poorly managed stress, they may listen more closely. Practically every physician and layperson knows now that stress can be dangerous. But once you say that there is an emotional component to poorly managed stress—such as out-of-control repressed anger or fear or anxiety—most people begin to get nervous.

QUESTION: Are you saying a wrong twist or turn is never the source of my muscle aches and pains?

ANSWER: Obviously, sometimes we hurt because of an acute injury to our body. It's certainly possible to strain a muscle because you've done something extraordinary. In that case, your pain should resolve in a couple of days.

But if the pain started after you did something that you've done a hundred times over, or if it goes on and on and on, don't make the mistake of blaming the twist or turn. I try to steer my patients away from the natural tendency to look for the mechanical or physical explanation, rather than looking at stress, pressure, and repressed emotions.

You may remember how, in my personal pain story, I woke up one morning with heel pain. My thought was, *What did I do last night—did I twist it wrong and now I just don't remember?* When that thought pattern starts, then bam! we miss the mind–body connection! We miss the opportunity to find the real cause for the pain—and get a permanent cure without swallowing a bunch of pills.

Frequently, patients have to get to the end of their rope: the pain has to become chronic with absolutely no pain relief or treatment in sight before they say, "You know what? Nothing else is working. Maybe I'll look for another answer." When they reach this point, they finally have the opportunity to find the real cause and the real cure.

QUESTION: You use the word *crutch* to describe some of the things I've been using, such as the heating pad and the magnet belt. But sometimes I really do feel better after using these things. Are you saying they don't help at all?

ANSWER: In AOS, part of the reason the muscles hurt is due to transient lack of blood flow and oxygen. Heating pads and magnet belts (supposedly) have the effect of helping blood flow to the muscle temporarily. Many times, you'll feel better for an hour or two.

But these devices are something I will not let my patients continue using. So if you have a magnetic belt, heating pad, or some similar gadget, throw it away! These crutches keep open the door to the "living room" physical explanations and physical answers to your pain. You have to shut that door completely!

Even though these things seem to help for a while, they will not help you one iota over the long haul. Instead, they keep you from getting better because they keep you from focusing on your repressed dangerous emotions as the exclusive treatment and answer for your pain.

QUESTION: Now that I see that my Perfectionism [or People-Pleasing, or Legalism, or another pain-prone personality trait] is contributing to my pain, do I need to change my personality?

ANSWER: It's absolutely true that different pain-prone personalities produce a lot of strong negative emotions. But it is your *repression* of these emotions that causes the pain, not the fact that they exist or that you possess a certain set of personality traits.

I don't think that people can change their basic personality. If you are born and bred a Perfectionist, you're always going to have tendencies in that direction. But I do think that when you are spiritually and emotionally healthy, your Perfectionist personality doesn't generate nearly the amount or degree of anger, pressure, or irritation it does when you're spiritually and emotionally unhealthy.

Rather than changing your personality, the challenge is to understand and acknowledge *how* your personality contributes to generating and repressing these dangerous emotions day in and day out. As you learn more about your personality—through such channels as pain talk and depth journaling—you'll become more skillful in identifying your emotions and expressing them appropriately.

I often suggest that my patients keep this short set of personality "marching orders" in mind:

- Recognize that you don't need to change your basic personality—just understand the strong negative emotions it causes!
- Become aware of how your personality creates those dangerous and strong negative emotions. Learn to recognize them as they occur.
- Keep a few basic questions in mind: *What pressure do I feel? Do I feel out of control or alone?* These are "gold mine" questions that will often help you keep up with your emotions and get to the source of any discomfort.

If you follow these marching orders closely and keep up with your spiritual and emotional health, you'll be less inclined to produce or repress the dangerous negative emotions that lay the groundwork for AOS pain and symptoms.

QUESTION: What about my X-rays, which show I have a herniated disk?

ANSWER: With each of my patients, I closely review X-rays as well as the recommendations from their local physicians. In these evaluations, I have found that herniated disks are very common in people over the age of forty. In fact, a *New England Journal of Medicine* study a few years ago said that more than 75 percent of people who have *never* had back pain still have herniated disks. The researchers also said that, given the high prevalence of disk bulges and protrusions, "the existence of low back pain and these X-ray 'abnormalities' may be coincidental."[1] In other words, the bulge or herniated disk is *normal* in most cases.

In my opinion, herniated disks are like wrinkles on your face. They are a normal part of aging and a normal part of wear and tear. But they do not cause pain in most cases. There is some evidence to suggest that when there are disk extrusions and shards of bone impinging on a nerve root, surgery is very successful. But most patients that I see with back pain and herniated disks do not have this finding on their MRI.

QUESTION: I get migraine headaches when I stop caffeine. What's that all about?

ANSWER: Caffeine withdrawal can certainly cause headaches. However, if you get chronic migraine headaches, caffeine is just the tip of the iceberg. AOS can produce vascular spasm leading to migraine headaches. Go through the 6-week program and lower your autonomic nervous system speedometer. Then you can drink moderate amounts of caffeine all you want.

QUESTION: I've had irritable bowel syndrome for years. There's some new pill out that is supposed to help. What do you think?

ANSWER: Irritable bowel syndrome (IBS) is caused by AOS. As I've said above, pills to prevent AOS symptoms, including IBS, are no cure. The real question is, *Why are my bowels so hyperactive—why do they squeeze so abnormally?* The pill won't answer those questions, and you'll be on it for life. I'm not against pills, but I would rather see you go through the Pain-Free for Life Program and find a lasting solution for your IBS.

QUESTION: What about lifts or arches in my shoes to relieve my back pain?

ANSWER: If one of your legs is a lot shorter than another, it's not a bad thing to wear orthotics. However, its been my experience that orthotics are *not* a solution to chronic back pain, fibromyalgia, or any of the other AOS symptoms I've described in this book. Lifts and arches don't help your muscles to relax when you have a mountain of repressed emotions driving your autonomic nervous system!

When I had my chronic back pain, I was told by one physician that my right leg was half an inch shorter than my left. I tried a set of thick shoe inserts for about a month, but that didn't help—and I finally took them out. My pain was from AOS, not from a short leg.

QUESTION: Should I switch to a hard mattress for my back pain?

ANSWER: I've never encountered a situation where hardness or softness of a mattress was a long-term factor in back pain. Sometimes you will sleep better for a few nights—but with AOS, the pain will soon come back on your new mattress! Instead, mattresses typically become a crutch that masks the real cause of the pain—buried emotions.

QUESTION: I have fibromyalgia and I'm afraid that the symptoms will get worse if I push too hard.

ANSWER: Remember, fibromyalgia is a type of AOS. Fibromyalgia (FM) patients commonly feel as though they are weaker and have more limitations than other people. This fear and concept of weakness plays a big role in the development of AOS fibromyalgia, and it also keeps the patients from getting better. So this fear of weakness must be overcome to become symptom-free.

I tell my FM patients that they must make up their mind that they're *not* weak. Part of their journaling should explore this whole concept of "weakness" and being frail. In their treatment plan, they need to exercise and play and stay out late if necessary—while confidently knowing that they are *normal* and *strong*—and they will get better.

QUESTION: I've heard that for back pain, doing stomach exercises to strengthen the abdominal muscles can help. What do you think?

ANSWER: I was also told this by a personal trainer I had when I was first trying to get out of pain. I tell patients quite plainly, "Strong abs are *not* the key to overcoming back pain." Doing stomach exercises may flatten your stomach and give you a hard six-pack. But even well-conditioned athletes who knock off hundreds of crunches at a time still end up with chronic back pain.

Just last month I had a patient in my office with chronic debilitating back pain—and his abs were worthy of a photo cover. The pain, in almost every case, is the work of the subconscious in activating the autonomic nervous system because of the dangerous levels of stuffed, repressed emotions. In my case, and in the case of hundreds of my patients who have *no* pain in their backs now—we don't have six-pack abs, believe me!

QUESTION: How about stretching exercises? Will they help my muscle aches?

ANSWER: Stretching exercises can increase your range of motion—an especially good fitness feature to foster as you grow older.[2] But several studies have shown that they have no effect in relieving back pain—or in preventing injury when they are used as a warm-up technique before a workout.[3] If you stretch because you enjoy it . . . or if you stretch before you exercise . . . or if you stretch to wake up in the morning—that's all great. However, if you stretch because you think you'll get muscle pain otherwise, the stretching is a crutch. In such a case, I would recommend that you stop stretching until your pain gets better with the Pain-Free for Life Program *alone*. Remember, any crutch will keep you from getting better if it serves to keep the door open to the physical explanations and treatment of your pain.

QUESTION: To protect my back, should I be careful about the way I lift things or the way I bend over?

ANSWER: Some argue that you can prevent back pain and injuries by not lifting more than about five pounds, or by bending at your knees rather than bending over with knees straight. However, I haven't found this to be true in practice or in my experience with AOS patients. Actually, a 1997 study of four thousand postal workers found the opposite.

Half of the workers were instructed to use their legs when they lifted and to follow other lifting techniques thought to put less pressure on the back. But the researchers determined that when compared with the workers who continued to lift the old way, the education program and proper lifting techniques didn't reduce the number of low back injuries; didn't reduce the cost per injury; didn't reduce the time lost from work; didn't reduce the rate of related musculoskeletal injuries; and didn't cut the rate of additional injuries after the subjects returned to work.[4]

QUESTION: My back and hip seem to hurt more when I drive or ride for long distances. I'm told it might be a problem with my pyraformis muscle.

ANSWER: Sitting in one position for long periods of time can produce cramping of muscles and joints—especially if you've got AOS. As a result, it's always advisable to take driving breaks as often as possible, and to move about every half hour or so if you're on a long plane or train trip. But the chances are, if you experience regular pain in your back or other locations on these trips, emotional stress and buried emotions are involved. Many of my patients with these travel pains find that their problem disappears—without reference to taking breaks or moving about—when they go through the 6-week program.

As for "pyraformis syndrome"—I think it is hogwash. The pyraformis muscle is about as big as your thumb and lies deep in your buttocks and hip area. Some doctors and physical therapists encourage patients to vigorously stretch out the pyraformis muscle in order to gain relief from lower back and hip pain. I have yet to find a patient who was cured from chronic back and hip pain by doing this.

QUESTION: Should I sleep on my stomach to relieve my pain?

ANSWER: That's another myth. Sleep on your stomach only if you like sleeping on your stomach. AOS and chronic back pain have nothing to do with sleeping positions.

A word about sleep: The subconscious mind is extremely active in your sleep—that's why we dream. Some of my patients experience more pain in the middle of the night during sleep. They get fooled into thinking it's the mattress or the pillow when in fact it's the activity of the subconscious mind. I recommend that AOS patients with this problem be sure to do the treatment steps later in the evening or just before bedtime.

QUESTION: To reduce my back pain, should I avoid swimming?

ANSWER: Another back pain myth is that arching your back, as you do when you swim the breaststroke, can cause chronic back pain. Although swimming is a wonderful exercise, it won't cure your back pain. But it will keep you in aerobic shape and burn those excess calories!

QUESTION: You've suggested that meditation can be an effective part of the Pain-Free for Life Program. I'm a Christian, and I'm wondering if that won't just get me into Eastern religious practices?

ANSWER: A common misconception, especially among many who are of the Christian faith, is that meditation is a practice confined to Eastern religions.

In fact, an important part of the prayer lives of King David and other writers of the Psalms was meditation on God's wonders, statutes, precepts, promises, and scriptures.[5] In other words, any Christian or Jew should feel comfortable meditating in the mode suggested by David and others, who focused on the content of the Scripture.

Meditation is as appropriate for Christians as for anyone else. In the Pain-Free Program, I talk about directed meditation—which is not a state of mind where you empty your mind and thoughts. Rather, you relax your body, breathe regularly and deeply to calm your mind, and direct your thoughts to things that are good and true and wonderful.

QUESTION: What's the best time to do the program?

ANSWER: Many of my patients have found that the best time— when they feel more relaxed and their minds can focus on subconscious emotions—is either early in the morning or just before bedtime. But there's certainly nothing wrong with going through your Pain-Free exercises at lunchtime or any other convenient hour. In my life, it seems easier to focus and relax before the stress of the day starts, or after the kids are down for bed.

Also, remember that the program has been designed for flexibility. So if you are riding for a while on a train or are stuck somewhere in an airport, pull out your writing pad or just sit quietly and begin the treatment plan. If you're in the middle of a stressful situation and you feel your back begin to tighten in response to dangerous emotions building—such as irritation or anger or fear—you can begin your pain talk or journaling right then if appropriate.

QUESTION: What if I don't get better with the 6-week program?

ANSWER: After I diagnose patients with AOS, I ask them to call me back after six weeks of following the program if they're not seeing significant improvement in their symptoms. About 80 percent will have wonderful improvement, and I won't hear from them except for a thank-you note. Of the ones who aren't improving, I'll ask questions to decide if they're just not understanding the treatment plan. Or I'll try to learn if they lack confidence in their diagnosis, or if they're just not insightful enough to find any significant repressed emotions.

If the problem is just a lack of understanding, I ask patients to watch the videotapes and review the material about AOS again. Most often, lack of confidence in the diagnosis is at issue; patients leave the door open to the physical explanations and physical answers. They just can't seem to get past the thought that their back has degenerative disks.

When this occurs, I'll review their case again to make sure we haven't left anything uncovered, and that I've done a thorough evaluation of their physical body and review of their labs and X-rays and haven't missed any true physical or structural problems. Many people will get better just by reading this book or listening to the *Freedom from Pain* videotapes. In some cases, however, people do need to come to the Brady Institute for Health for assurance and confidence in a diagnosis of AOS.

For those who understand the treatment plan and have confidence in the AOS diagnosis—but just can't seem to find many charged buried emotions—I'll refer them to a psychologist.

QUESTION: How is the Pain-Free for Life treatment of Autonomic Overload Syndrome (AOS) different from TMS?

ANSWER: More than twenty years ago, Dr. John Sarno coined the term *Tension Myositis Syndrome* (*TMS*) in reference to a group of disorders caused by repressed anger and rage in the unconscious mind. *Tension* refers to psychological tension. *Myositis* refers to muscle inflammation (though Sarno himself later understood that there was no actual inflammation of the muscle). The TMS treatment plan emphasizes knowledge of the unconscious process.

Dr. Sarno and the TMS concepts published in medical literature were influential in my early understanding of mind–body interactions. But more recently I have formulated the Autonomic Overload Syndrome concept to encompass both the latest mind–body research by other scientists and also distinctive findings in my own research and clinical practice, including the importance of spiritual dysfunction as a source of chronic pain.

More recent medical research has confirmed that dangerous levels of stress and emotions associated with stress can lead to overload and overactivation of the autonomic nervous system. Dr. Bruce S. McEwen and others have published extensively in the medical literature regarding the dangerous physical effects of autonomic overload (or, as McEwen calls it, allostatic overload).

In my own personal and clinical experience, *AOS* has emerged as an accurate umbrella term to cover the mind–body–spirit sources of many types of chronic pain, and also to point toward the mind–body–spirit solutions and treatments that are described in this book. Over several years, I have formulated a step-by-step treatment plan that identifies subconscious repressed emotions and reverses AOS symptoms. My mind–body–spirit techniques, which have provided significant help with AOS, include what I call pain talk, pain visualization, and directed meditation. Finally, I've relied heavily on recent medical research to develop the critically successful treatment step that I have termed depth journaling.

In short, the Pain-Free for Life Program has been built on the insights and research of many scientists and physicians. But I trust that we have not reached the end of the line in this process. It is my hope that others will build on my program in ways that have yet to be explored.

QUESTION: When do I need to see a psychologist?

ANSWER: About 10 to 15 percent of AOS patients do not experience significant pain relief after six to eight weeks. In these cases, I will ask them to seek the help of a trained mental health professional. The object of this is to help patients discover the repressed dangerous emotions that they're unable to find themselves.

It's best if the psychologist is trained in psychoanalytical techniques, which involve digging deep into the subconscious to find repressed emotions. If the specialist is a behavioral psychologist, he or she may be able to help you reframe your situation and develop coping mechanisms. But those with this background are generally not experts at asking questions to dig up what you've so successfully buried.

QUESTION: Is there any typical course for AOS recovery from chronic pain?

ANSWER: No recovery experience is the same. However, it is not uncommon in AOS recovery for patients to experience a recovery sequence like this:

* Your chronic pain symptoms actually get *worse* after you recognize some of the dangerous repressed emotions.

- You take a few steps forward and get relief, but then take one step back and lose ground to the pain. When you're getting close to some significant repressed emotions, you can expect symptoms to increase. But don't give up—they *will* go away if you continue!
- Your AOS symptoms move around when you eliminate AOS symptoms from one part of the body—the back pain, for instance, may go away, then pop up again elsewhere, such as in a headache or a bout of irritable bowel syndrome.
- About 10 percent of AOS patients recover in less than a week—after an aha moment when they perceive that the source of the pain is repressed emotions, not a structural problem. But most patients have to go through the 6-week program to experience significant relief.

QUESTION: How long do I have to stay on the program after I'm cured?

ANSWER: Some patients go through the program and never have a pain or twinge again. However, because you'll keep your anger-generating personality with you, it's common to experience a few symptoms here and there. If you don't keep up with your emotions, you can certainly experience AOS symptoms again.

I haven't had back pain in more than seven years. But two or three times a year, I might begin feeling a mild muscle tightness, or the beginnings of a bout of irritable bowel. The symptoms serve as a reminder to me: *Oh yeah, I really do feel irritated and under a lot of pressure, and I haven't given it any thought for months.*

I think the best approach is to assume that you should *remain alert* to future AOS symptoms produced by your subconscious mind. Also, remember that the more time you spend consciously thinking about your dangerous emotions and about managing them constructively, the less chance there is that you'll ever have AOS symptoms again.

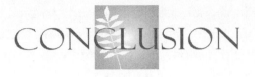

CONCLUSION

FROM PAIN TO WHOLENESS

In life, there are a few pivotal turns—moments when life changes one way or another, and it will never be the same. For me, getting out of pain was one of those turns. When I look back, slowly but surely, the back pain had consumed my thoughts, my activities, my family, my happiness—my life.

Those of you in pain know exactly what I'm talking about: If your mind has a thousand thoughts each day, five hundred of them are taken up with pain. I remember one evening sitting in a booth at a local restaurant. I think I asked my wife to repeat the story she was telling about three times. The thought went through my mind: *I can't do it—I can't even pay attention and listen to my wife because all I can think about is how uncomfortable this booth feels and how painful my back is.*

Almost every waking hour I was thinking about what could make my pain feel better (sit a certain way, bend over a little, stand up), or when it would be time to take my next round of pills to take the edge off.

Abby was our only child back then. I remember when she would hold her arms in the air, asking for Daddy to pick her up. Sometimes, I'd grit my teeth, bend over, and endure the pain. But most of the time I would just take her hand and walk, hoping that would be enough. I had become a slave to pain.

You may not think it's possible, but once you're out of pain, it's hard to remember what life was like when the pain was there. Also, it's hard to believe how much you can experience *now* that you had no hope for *then*.

I was thinking about that very thing one evening a few weeks ago when I was relaxing with my wife, Pamela. We had just built a cabin in the northern Georgia mountains, and we were there taking our summer family vacation. One evening before bed we were talking about the day, and it struck me how many things we had enjoyed just in the past six hours—things that years ago I thought I'd never enjoy again.

Earlier that evening my wife, our four girls, and I had taken a short hike down an old logging trail around the mountain. The road isn't used anymore, but the trail is perfect for a hike down to a little tiny creek. The walk began with everyone jumping, dancing, and talking up a storm. After a few minutes, Hannah, the little one (age two), needed to be held, so I held her in my left arm and carried all the walking sticks and just-picked flowers in my right hand.

Halfway down the trail, we came across a tree that had fallen; it had landed against the bank and come to rest in a horizontal position about three feet above the ground. Of course, to my daughters it looked like a perfect balance beam, so I lifted each of them up to try her shot at tree gymnastics. Could I still do a skin-the-cat? they asked. To my surprise, I still could.

The pinnacle of the hike came when we got to the little creek. We had to go down an awkward, slippery embankment to get there. I went first—and slipped and twisted and fell. But I got back up quickly to help the five ladies. Lydia and Sarah just wanted to jump into my arms instead of braving the bank—so they leaped three feet or so right into my grasp.

We then walked to the little creek where everyone wanted to take a drink, but the bank was slippery and unstable. So one by one, I took turns holding Abigail (age eight), Lydia (five), Sarah (four), and little Hannah *straight out* like an ironing board, slowly lowering each down to the water where she took a sip with her hand. Then it was straight up into my arms, and a little toss up to the top of the creekbank.

No problem, no pain, I'm not even thinking about it.

On the walk home, we threw rocks, picked up branches and swatted the briars as though we were mowing the lawn. Finally, both Sarah and Lydia decided they were too tired to walk back. So it was up on my shoulders with Lydia, and in my left arm with Sarah. Pamela had Hannah, the water jugs, the flowers, and a multitude of other things.

When we got back to the cabin, Pamela and the kids got ready for supper while I stayed out in the backyard, getting ready for the evening's big event—the bonfire. The first thing for me to do was to make some stools to sit on, so I got the chain saw going and cut a large fallen tree into eight or ten sections of about twenty-four inches each. Set upright, the sections made great fire-pit stools. The fire pit was about twenty yards away, and the stools each weighed about thirty pounds. But instead of walking up and down the hill, I tossed each tree section as far and high as I could and let gravity take it down to the flat area in the yard.

Next, it was time to collect the firewood: small twigs first; middle-size branches next; then large logs, the kind that burn for a couple of hours. Then we all laughed and played our new favorite game, You're On the Stump, where Dad points the stick to someone and says, "You're next on the stump." When you're on the stump, you've got to either sing or tell a story.

All the time, Pamela and I were roasting marshmallows and making s'mores for the kids.

After the bonfire, it was up the hill to the cabin for baths before bedtime. Of course, I got to tote the food and dirty shoes and a couple of kids under my arms. No problem, no pain, I'm not even thinking about it.

After baths—no easy trick lifting up kids in and out of the bathtub—it was time for a little rumbling around on the floor before bed. So I tickled and rolled and tossed kids all over the place while Lydia and Abigail got on my back and practiced riding me like a horse. Finally, bedtime arrived, with stories and sleep.

Of course, after the kids were down, the day didn't end. Pamela and I began the cleanup routine—bending, lifting, stooping, twisting, and everything else you do every day without thinking about it. But after the cleaning came the best part—relaxing and talking to my bride.

It's amazing how great it is to be able to focus, ask questions, and listen. I'm so thankful to be able to enjoy my wife and kids now; it seems easy and natural. I don't even think about how hard life used to be anymore, because life changed and I'm out of pain—for good.

Now, most books begin with a dedication, and mine is no different. But I want to give it to you again, because if you're suffering from pain, it's my deepest hope for you:

To those who are in Pain.
To those who have followed all the "right" medical paths—
but still continue to suffer.
To those who have lost hope
because "life" has been replaced with Pain.
I was there . . . and now I'm Pain-Free.
Take courage;
there is HOPE!

ENDNOTES

CHAPTER 3

[1]Kolata, G. "Healing a Bad Back Is Often an Effort in Painful Futility." *New York Times,* February 9, 2004. www.nytimes.com.

[2]National Institute of Neurological Disorders and Stroke (NINDS). "Low Back Pain Fact Sheet." www.ninds.nih.gov.

[3]www.mayoclinic.com/invoke.cfm?id=PN00036. See also *Journal of the American Academy of Nurse Practitioners* 15 (Supplement 12), December 2003: 3–9; *Langenbecks Archives of Surgery* 389 (4), August 2004: 237–43; *Journal of Head Trauma Rehabilitation* 19 (1), January–February 2004: 2–9.

[4]Ibid.

[5]"Fibromyalgia." www.MayoClinic.com.

[6]Hadhazy, V., Ezzo, J., and Creamer, P. "Mind-Body Therapies for the Treatment of Fibromyalgia: A Systematic Review." *Journal of Rheumatology* 27, 2000: 2911–8; Berman, B., and Swyers, J. "Complementary Medicine Treatments for Fibromyalgia Syndrome." *Clinical Rheumatology* 13, 1999: 487–92.

[7]Loew, T., and Sohn, R. "Functional Relaxation as a Somatopsychothera-

peutic Intervention: A Prospective Controlled Study." *Alternative Ther. Health Med.* 6, 2000: 70–5.

[8]Mayo Clinic staff. "Migraine." www.MayoClinic.com.

[9]Mayo Clinic staff. "Tension-Type Headache." www.MayoClinic.com.

[10]Horwitz, B. J., and Fisher, R. S. "The Irritable Bowel Syndrome." *New England Journal of Medicine* 344, June 14, 2001: 1846–50.

[11]Leclerc, A., and Niedhammer, I. "One-Year Predictive Factors for Various Aspects of Neck Disorders." *Spine* 24, 1999: 1455–62.

[12]Lundberg, U., and Dohns, I. E. "Psychophysiological Stress Responses, Muscle Tension, and Neck and Shoulder Pain Among Supermarket Cashiers." *Journal of Occupational Health and Psychology* 4, 1999: 245–55.

[13]Bilkis, M., and Mark, K. "Mind-Body Medicine: Practical Applications in Dermatology." *Archives of Dermatology* 134, 1998: 1437–41; Cohen, F., Kemeny, M. E., and Kearney, K. A. "Persistent Stress as a Predictor of Genital Herpes Recurrence." *Archives of Internal Medicine* 159, 1999: 2430–6.

[14]*Archives of Dermatology* 1998.

[15]Zinn, J. K. "Mindfulness Meditation." 1998.

CHAPTER 4

[1]McEwen, B. S. "Protection and Damage from Acute and Chronic Stress: Allostasis and Allostatic Overload and Relevance to the Pathophysiology of Psychiatric Disorders." *Annals of the New York Academy of Sciences* 1032, 2004: 1–7.

[2]*Mayo Clinic Proceedings,* February 2000.

[3]*New England Journal of Medicine* 352, February 10, 2005: 539–48.

[4]*New York Times,* February 10, 2005. www.nytimes.com.

[5]Leor, J., Poole, W., and Kloner, R. "Sudden Cardiac Death Triggered by an Earthquake." *New England Journal of Medicine* 334, 1996: 413–9.

[6]Galea, S., et al. "Psychological Sequelae of the September 11 Terrorist Attacks in New York City." *New England Journal of Medicine* 346, 2002: 982–7.

[7]Larsson, R., Oberg, P. A., and Larsson, S. E. "Changes of Trapezius Muscle Blood Flow and Electromyography in Chronic Neck Pain Due to Trapezius Myalgia." *Pain* 79, 1999: 45–50; Larsson, R., Cai, H., Zhang, B. Q., Oberg, P. A., and Larsson, S. E. "Visualization of Chronic Neck–Shoulder Pain: Impaired Microcirculation in the Upper Trapezius Muscle in Chronic Cervico-Brachial Pain." *Occupational Medicine* (London) 48, 1998: 189–94.

[8]Freud, S., from second of a series of five lectures delivered in 1909 at Clark University, Worcester, Massachusetts, on the origin and development of psychoanalysis.

CHAPTER 6

[1] Mitka, M. "Getting Religion Seen as Help in Being Well." *Journal of the American Medical Association* 280, 1998: 1896–7.

[2] *American Heart Journal* 142, November 2001.

[3]Koenig, H. G., McCullough, M. E., and Larson, D. B., eds. *Handbook of Religion and Health*. Oxford: Oxford University Press, 2001.

[4]Stanford University Medical Center, press release, May 10, 2005. http://med-www.stanford.edu/MedCenter/MedSchool.

[5]Koenig, McCullough, and Larson, eds. *Handbook:* 357.

[6]Kaplan, R. M., ed. "Special Issue: Spirituality, Religiousness, and Health: From Research to Clinical Practice." *Annals of Behavioral Medicine* 24 (1), 2002; Benson, H., and Proctor, W. *The Breakout Principle*. New York: Scribner, 2003, 2004: 257ff.

[7]Anandarajah, G., and Hight, E. "Spirituality and Medical Practice: Using the HOPE Questions as a Practical Tool for Spiritual Assessment." *American Family Physician* 63, 2001: 81–9.

[8]Ibid.

CHAPTER 7

[1]Benson, H., and Proctor, W. *The Breakout Principle*. New York: Scribner, 2003, 2004: 223–4.

[2]Ibid., 15. See also Adams, F. *The Genuine Works of Hippocrates*. London:

Syndenham Society, 1849; Castiglioni, A. *A History of Medicine,* translated by E. B. Krimbhaar. New York: Alfred A. Knopf, 1941.

[3]Sarno, J. E. *Healing Back Pain.* New York: Warner Books, 1991: 132.

[4]See Pert, C. B. *Molecules of Emotion.* New York: Simon & Schuster, 1997, 1999: 18, 304; Benson, H. *Timeless Healing.* New York: Simon & Schuster, 1996, 1997: 67–8, 94.

[5]Eisenberg, D. M., and Kessler, R. C. "Unconventional Medicine in the United States: Prevalence, Costs, and Patterns of Use." *New England Journal of Medicine* 328, 1993: 246–52; Sullivan, M. "Integrative Medicine: Making It Work for You." *Emergency Medicine,* October 2000: 76–82.

[6]See the excellent historical survey by Taylor, E. I. *Harvard Medical Alumni Bulletin,* winter 2000: 40–7. Some facts in the subsequent discussion, which relate to the Harvard background, have been drawn from his article.

[7]Benson, H. *The Relaxation Response.* New York: Morrow, 1975; Benson, H., Beary, J. F., and Carol, M. P. *Psychiatry* 37, 1974: 37–46; Beary, J. F., and Benson, H. *Psychosomatic Medicine* 36, 1974: 115–20.

[8]Pert, C. B. *Molecules of Emotion.* For sections of her book that pertain to the following discussion, see pp. 131, 146, 147, 179, 187, 189, 242, 243. See also her article in the *Journal of Immunology* 135 (2), August 1985.

[9]Sarno, J. E. *Healing Back Pain.* New York: Warner Books, 1991: ix; see also Sarno, J. E. *The Mindbody Prescription.* New York: Warner Books, 1998, 1999: xvii.

CHAPTER 9

[1]Smyth, J. M., et al. "Effects of Writing About Stressful Experiences on Symptom Reduction in Patients with Asthma or Rheumatoid Arthritis." *Journal of the American Medical Association* 281, April 14, 1999: 1304–9.

[2]Holmes, T., and Rahe, R. "Social Readjustment Rating Scale." *Journal of Psychosomatic Research* 2, 1967: 214.

CHAPTER 11

[1]Magni, G., et al. "Chronic Musculoskeletal Pain and Depressive Symptoms in the National Health and Nutrition Examination. I. Epidemiologic Follow-up Study." *Pain* 53, 1993: 163–8.

[2]Atkinson, et al. "Prevalence, Onset and Risk of Psychiatric Disorders in Men with Chronic Low Back Pain: A Controlled Study." *Pain* 45, 1991: 111–21; Katon, W. and M. Sullivan. "Depression and a Chronic Medical Illness." *Journal of Clinical Psychiatry* 150 (Supplement), 1990: 3–11; Sullivan, M. and W. Katon. "Somatization: The Path between Distress and Somatic Symptoms." *American Pain Society Journal* 2, 1993: 141–9; Sullivan, M. et al. "The Treatment of Depression in Chronic Low Back Pain: Review and Recommendations." *Pain* 50, 1992: 5–13. See also Clark, M., "Chronic Pain, Depression and Antidepressants: Issues and Relationships." Johns Hopkins Arthritis. www.hopkins-arthritis.som.jhmi.edu; "Depression Statistics Information." www.add-adhd-help-center.com; "About Depression." www.lexapro.com; National Mental Health Association. "Dysthmia." www.nmha.org.

CHAPTER 12

[1] *New England Journal of Medicine* 331, 1994: 69–73.

[2] *Archives of Physical and Medical Rehabilitation* 69, 1988: 268–72.

[3] Cooper, H. H. *Regaining the Power of Youth at Any Age*. Nashville: Thomas Nelson, 1987: 46.

[4] *New England Journal of Medicine,* July 1997.

[5]See especially Psalm 1:2 and all of Psalm 119.

ABOUT THE AUTHORS

SCOTT BRADY, MD, is the founder and director of the Brady Institute for Health at Florida Hospital in Celebration, Florida. He received his medical training at the Wake Forest University School of Medicine, after which he completed his residency and board certification in Internal Medicine in Orlando, Florida. Dr. Brady has practiced emergency and urgent care medicine throughout central Florida for more than fifteen years. He is the administrator and senior medical director of Florida Hospital's sixteen Centra Care urgent care centers. Dr. Brady is also the medical director of Get Healthy, Florida, which has worked with Florida Hospital Centra Care and the Florida Department of Health to distribute more than one hundred thousand doses of influenza vaccine throughout central Florida.

An accomplished communicator and health educator, Dr. Brady is a frequent guest lecturer to physicians, churches, and patient groups on topics including fibromyalgia, chronic back pain, mind–body–spirit disorders, the stress response, and mind–body medicine. He is frequently interviewed as a medical expert on various health topics by local television and radio.

In addition to his medical practice in Florida, Dr. Brady has traveled extensively, helping treat patients in hospitals and clinics in underserved areas including Zaire, Swaziland, Kenya, Brazil, and Ukraine. Dr. Brady and his wife, Pamela, live in Orlando along with their four daughters, Abigail Grace, Lydia Grace, Sarah Grace, and Hannah Grace—or, as they call it, the Brady Sisters Fun Club.

WILLIAM PROCTOR, a graduate of Harvard College and Law School, has written more than eighty books, including several international best sellers on medical topics. His books have been translated into more than forty languages and have sold more than ten million copies. More information on his writing and speaking activities is available on his Web site, www.WilliamProctor.com.

The Brady Institute for Health (www.BradyInstitute.com)

Dr. Scott Brady established the Brady Institute for Health on the premises of Florida Hospital–Celebration. The institute is dedicated to mind–body–spirit evaluation and treatment of patients who suffer from AOS.

Patients from all over the world have come to the Brady Institute for Health for relief of AOS chronic pain. Several years ago, in recognition that such travel can be prohibitive for some, Dr. Brady put his lectures on video in a three-tape series, *Freedom from Pain*. This video series is also available at www.BradyInstitute.com.

In tape 1, you'll learn about Autonomic Overload Syndrome and how your thoughts, stress, pressure, and repressed emotions can affect your physical body with abnormal changes to the nervous system and muscles. You'll be introduced to the subconscious mind and discover how it directs the autonomic nervous system and the stress response to produce painful AOS symptoms.

Tape 2 will tell you more about the true culprit for AOS: critical levels of repressed emotions and stress. You'll learn about a few common personalities of people who get AOS and about the steps you can take to stop AOS symptoms altogether.

Tape 3 focuses on the mind–body–spirit connection. In this lecture, Dr. Brady teaches you the important role of spiritual health in the maintenance of the pain-free life. You'll learn how psychological health, physical health, and spiritual health all interact, and how spiritual health helps keep daily stress and pressures from causing AOS symptoms.

Dr. Brady would love to hear from you. If you would like to share your personal story of starting your Pain-Free life, please write to Dr. Brady at:

Scott Brady, MD
c/o Florida Hospital Centra Care
901 North Lake Destiny Road
Suite 400
Maitland, FL 32751

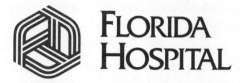

FLORIDA HOSPITAL

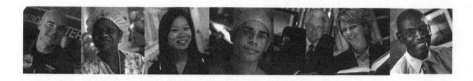

ABOUT FLORIDA HOSPITAL
AMERICA'S TRUSTED LEADER FOR HEALTH AND HEALING

For nearly a hundred years, the mission of Florida Hospital has been to help patients, guests, and friends achieve whole-person health and healing. With seven hospital campuses and fourteen walk-in medical centers, Florida Hospital cares for nearly one million patients every year.

More than a decade ago, Florida Hospital began working with the Disney Corporation to create a groundbreaking facility that would showcase the model of health care for the twenty-first century and stay on the cutting edge of medical technology as it develops. Working with a team of medical experts, industry leaders, and health care futurists, we designed and built a whole-person health hospital named Celebration Health located in Disney's town of Celebration, Florida. Since opening its doors in 1997, Celebration Health has been awarded the Premier Patient Services Innovator Award as "The Model for Healthcare Delivery in the 21st Century."

When Dr. Lydia Parmele, the first female physician in the state of Florida, and her medical team opened our first health care facility in 1908, their goal was to create a healing environment where they not only treated illness, but also provided the support and education necessary to help patients achieve whole-person health mentally, physically, spiritually, emotionally, and socially.

The lifestyle advocated by its founders remains central to Florida Hospital. Patients are taught how to reduce the risk of disease through healthy lifestyle choices and the use of natural remedies such as fresh air, sunshine, water, rest, nutrition, exercise, outlook, faith, and interpersonal relationships.

Today, Florida Hospital:

- Is ranked number one in the nation for inpatient admissions by the American Hospital Association.
- Is the largest provider of Medicare services in the country.
- Performs the most heart procedures each year, making it the number one hospital fighting America's number one killer—heart disease.
- Operates many nationally recognized centers of excellence, including cardiology, cancer, orthopedics, neurology and neurosurgery, digestive disorders, and minimally invasive surgery.
- Is one of the "Top 10 Best Places in the Country to Have a Baby" according to *Fit Pregnancy* magazine.

For more information about Florida Hospital and its whole-person health products, including books, music, videos, conferences, seminars, and other resources, please contact:

FLORIDA HOSPITAL PUBLISHING
683 Winyah Drive
Orlando, FL 32803
Phone: 407-303-7711
Fax: 407-303-1818
E-mail: healthproducts@flhosp.org
www.floridahospital.com
www.creationhealth.com

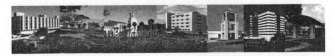

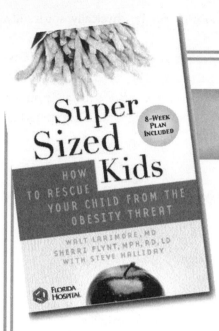
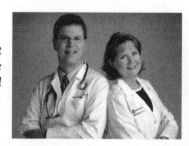